Emotions and reflexivity in Health and Social Care Field Research

Helen T. Allan • Anne Arber
Editors

Emotions and reflexivity in Health and Social Care Field Research

palgrave
macmillan

Editors
Helen T. Allan
Middlesex University
London, UK

Anne Arber
University of Surrey
Guildford, UK

ISBN 978-3-319-65502-4 ISBN 978-3-319-65503-1 (eBook)
https://doi.org/10.1007/978-3-319-65503-1

Library of Congress Control Number: 2017956091

Cover illustration: PhotoAlto sas / Alamy Stock Photo

Printed on acid-free paper

This Palgrave Macmillan imprint is published by Springer Nature
The registered company is Springer International Publishing AG
The registered company address is: Gewerbestrasse 11, 6330 Cham, Switzerland

Helen would like to dedicate this book to her students who have been a delight to supervise (mainly) and provided her with huge learning opportunities over the years. Anne would like to dedicate this book to all the healthcare practitioners who have supported her and to her family Mick, Ruth, Ian and Morgane.

Foreword

In this book, Helen Allan and Anne Arber bring together a unique mix of their own and their students' experiences of doctoral research and supervision. They combine accounts of the student and supervisor journey to tell a story in which emotions, reflexivity and relationships play a key role in the production of new knowledge. They highlight the importance of relationships at all levels and challenge us to see our emotions as a resource rather than a risk as they take us behind metaphorical closed doors to reveal the crafting of a thesis by supervisor and student. We are given a lexicon with which to recognise and name emotions as a part of the supervision process rather than hide them. Reflexivity is the essential tool which enables us to do this as illustrated by the studies presented in the book. Each chapter encourages the reader to consider emotions as a topic for research, as data and as an empirical tool which involves reflexivity as 'a reaction to an emotion'.

The process of supervision, being in the field, data collection and analysis create a matrix of relationships between student and supervisor; researcher and participants; data collection and analysis; practitioner-researcher, which enrich and enhance the research. As all authors reflect 'the practitioner-researcher moves between the different ways of being in a more dynamic way' while for Helen and Anne 'guiding students to learn how to process feelings and then with those feelings as students learn more and more expertly to process their fieldwork experiences and to debrief events' are at the very heart of supervision. We are also reminded how important it is to learn to gauge the level of emotional engagement with research participants. These insights highlight the book's importance in naming and making visible the tacit skills involved in supervising and undertaking doctoral research. In this regard, Sarah Li reminds us of the importance of keeping a research diary in which thoughts and feelings can be documented and shared between supervisor and student. I was also reminded of the sociologist C. Wright Mills' advice to beginning students that by 'keeping an adequate file and thus developing self-reflective habits you learn how to keep your inner world awake' (Wright Mills, 1959: 197). He also urges students to 'build up the habit of writing' and use 'observation and daily experience'.

C. Wright Mills' view that 'social science is the practice of a craft' is apparent in the range of topics presented in the book and the juxtaposition of theory, methodology and more specifically phenomenology, psychoanalysis and ethnography to illuminate emotions. One of the ways students learn to practise their craft is through the development of researcher-participant relationships which take many forms during the doctoral process. For example, Nicola Ayers discusses the effects of working in a different culture and country; Kit Tapson describes researching marginalised and difficult-to-reach young people and the need to sensitively manage their anxiety and aggression during data collection while being mindful of her own safety; Tam Cane tells us that research with participants with HIV-related infertility generated tensions associated with being both a researcher and a social worker as well as her personal concern about parenthood; for Ginny Mounce, it was the need to have 'sustained involvement' over time with her participants which presented her with emotional challenges. Nicola and Tam's examples suggest the emotionally laden reasons why particular study topics are chosen in the first place while Kit and Ginny's examples draw attention to the 'emotional labour' required to navigate their way through sensitive field relations.

The book's success is its ability to give new insights and encourage reflection and critique of past and present research on emotions. Emotional labour is just one example of a theory the authors consider. First described by sociologist Arlie Hochschild in 1983 to describe 'people work' in the service sector, emotional labour still remains an intriguing and innovative middle-range theory for naming emotions and the processes involved in managing them. In the intervening decades, emotional labour has been subject to scrutiny and critical refinement resulting in a variety of interpretations and applications to nursing, midwifery, medicine, social and care work. Reading Nicola's, Tam's, Kit's and Ginny's accounts evoked memories of my own doctoral research, and early days in the field when during interviews with students, I first experienced care as labour through the language they used and the feelings they expressed which conveyed a sense of the sheer emotional work required.

One student explained that she came into nursing to care for people. She said: 'I expected to care for them in pain and when they were dying. What I didn't expect was that the system doesn't always let me do it in the way I want to'. Students were more likely to feel this way on wards where the sisters managed hierarchically and produced negative emotional labour, which made them feel frightened, anxious and stressed.

The ward sister/charge nurse was identified as the key person who set the emotional tone for the caring climate on the ward. As one student explained: '[I]f sister cares then I don't need to take the whole caring attitude of the whole ward on my shoulders' (Smith, 1992, 2012).

Helen and Anne flag up 'the difficulty of being alive to emotions in the field' and in particular those associated with 'sorrow, loss, disappointment or grief' all of which are reflected in the above accounts. In recent years, psychologists have suggested that a diverse array of emotions can be reduced to four essentials, which include happiness, sadness, fear/surprise, anger/disgust (Jack et al., 2016). Naming happiness is a useful reminder that emotions may not always be 'burdensome'.

To conclude, I refer to the classic anthropological novel *Return to Laughter* (Bowen, 1954), which I read over 33 years ago while undertaking my doctoral fieldwork. The novel came to mind while reflecting on and writing this foreword. The author lived for a year in a remote Nigerian village when she was a young anthropologist and ethnographer. She describes the anxieties and dilemmas, but also the enriching experience of living in two cultures, the isolation of being the only European, learning a new language, acknowledging social mores and developing the sensitivity required to sustain good field relations while maintaining her boundaries to enable her to collect data, write field notes and conduct analysis. The author (Laura Bohannan) wrote under a 'nom de plume'

(Elenore Smith Bowen) to protect her academic credibility (given the low regard, such a qualitative account would have had within the academic community of the time) and to protect her participants. Bowen's story further highlights the importance of taking gender, race and ethnicity into account while in the field.

When asking myself why I remembered *Return to Laughter* after more than 30 years, I attributed this to the powerful emotional resonances I experienced when reading Helen, Anne, Sarah, Nicola, Kit, Tam and Ginny's chapters, stimulating me to reflect and remember a book I had read so long ago. This is a sign Helen, Anne and their co-authors have written not only a good book but an invaluable book which recognises and uses emotions and reflexivity to practise the craft of health and social research. It is also a book about the doctoral journey and supporting supervisors and students to pass on their craft and their knowledge to future generations

Nursing Studies
University of Edinburgh,
Edinburgh, UK
July 8, 2017

Pam Smith

References

Bowen, S. E. (1954). *Return to laughter*. New York: Harper and Brothers.

Hochschild, A. R. (1983). *The managed heart: The commercialisation of human feeling*. Berkeley, CA: University of California Press.

Jack, R. E., Sun, W., Delis, I., Garrod, O. G. B., & Schyns, P. G. (2016). Four not six: Revealing culturally common facial expressions of emotions. *Journal of Experimental Psychology: General, 145*(6), 708–730.

Mills, C. W. (1959). *The sociological imagination*: Appendix on Intellectual Craftsmanship. Oxford: Oxford University Press.

Smith, P. (1992). *The emotional labour of nursing: How nurses care*. Basingstoke: Palgrave Macmillan.

Smith, P. (2012). *The emotional labour of nursing revisited: Can nurses still care?* (2nd ed.). Basingstoke: Palgrave Macmillan.

Preface

As contributors and editors to this book, we believe that emotions and reflexivity are integrally linked as emotions motivate us to reflexivity; this is a central theme of the book. This book is a collaboration between academic supervisors (the editors) and some of our doctoral students. We, alongside Sarah Li, are experienced ethnographers/Ph.D. supervisors and have (over the years) spent many hours discussing reflexivity and emotions in research between ourselves and with our students in health and social care settings.

We've written this book for doctoral students and their supervisors and deliberately chosen to incorporate both sides of the doctoral supervision relationship: both students and supervisors. The book draws on our work as ethnographers interested in emotions when conducting fieldwork. The first chapter is written as an introduction to reflexivity and emotions. Chapter 2 identifies a natural history of a Ph.D. study with an introduction to reflexivity in the researcher and supervisor relationship during an ethnography conducted in palliative care settings in the UK. Chapters 3 and 4 are ethnographies conducted in the fertility clinic discussing hidden emotions and palliative care settings discussing the dual identity as a researcher and a practitioner and the challenges that brings to field work. Chapters 5–8 are written by recently completed Ph.D. students. All chapters draw on field work undertaken as a part of doctoral studies where contributors draw on emotional reflexivity at key points in the research journey and during supervision. Chapter 9 pulls things together and has some final suggestions on how to engage with emotional reflexivity in health and social care field research.

Having chapters in different areas of practice, including mental health, young people and bullying, palliative care, infertility, ethnography both at home and overseas allows us to cover a wide range of methodological issues relevant to an emotional reflexivity. For example, the role of the practitioner in (ethnographic) fieldwork, insider/outsider issues experienced during fieldwork, issues of access to hard-to-reach groups, the body and technology, the collision of roles of researcher/professional/practitioner/personal during fieldwork and leaving the field.

The book is organized into chapters but we recommend you read it as a whole as there are shared ideas which take shape through each of the chapters as authors add their own meaning to a discussion of emotions and reflexivity in healthcare research. We have also given our book an educational focus, by which we mean a focus on the process of learning through emotions as a researcher. We all use field research methodology (ethnography, observational research) as a way into emotional reflexivity. This book is written with the needs of postgraduates and researchers in mind.

We would like to acknowledge the contributions of all our students whose learning we have implicitly drawn on to write this book and our own supervisors who supported us on our doctoral journey. They are Jan Savage, Clive Seale and Pam Smith.

London, UK
June 2017

Helen T. Allan
Anne Arber

Contents

About the Editors

Helen T. Allan is Professor of Nursing at Middlesex University, London, UK. Helen has held Chairs at the Universities of Surrey and York. Helen has a clinical background in acute care and a BSc Sociology from the London School of Economics. Helen worked as a nurse teacher for a number of years while completing her Ph.D. in Nursing part time at Manchester University. She has supervised research students since 2002. Helen uses feminist research methodologies, qualitative and mixed methods and action research. Her research and practice interests include nursing education, practice learning, healthcare organizations and reproductive technologies, women's health and midwifery.

Anne Arber is Senior Lecturer in Cancer and Palliative Care at the University of Surrey. She has a clinical background in cancer nursing. Her research focuses on supportive care for patients with cancer and their carers, including support for family members and symptom support using e-health. She is an experienced Ph.D. supervisor and combines research and teaching as part of her role. She has research expertise in discourse analysis, ethnography and mixed methods research. She is a trainer in Advanced Communication Skills and has been invited to run workshops in advanced communication in the UK and Europe.

1

Introduction

Helen T. Allan and Anne Arber

Introduction

This book is about researchers' experiences of doing emotional reflexivity in health and social care settings. While reflexivity has become an integral part of research practice and supervision (Seale, 1999) and a defining feature of qualitative research (Finlay, 2002), questions remain about how to go about doing emotional reflexivity. Researchers in health and social care settings like other researchers are part of the social worlds they study. They may have multiple identities such as practitioner, counsellor as well as researcher, and they may be motivated to research in certain areas because they have experienced illness themselves. Researchers' experiences, interactions, emotional involvement and reflections on what they observe form parts of the research process, data analysis and the written account, and are the means by which knowledge is developed (Hammersley, 1992).

H.T. Allan (✉)
Department of Adult, Child, Midwifery, Middlesex University, London, UK

A. Arber
University of Surrey, Guildford, UK

H.T. Allan, A. Arber (eds.), *Emotions and reflexivity in Health and Social Care Field Research*, https://doi.org/10.1007/978-3-319-65503-1_1

Reflexivity in ethnography and field research helps researchers to integrate social reality in the sense that, in being reflexive, the experience of the researcher is acknowledged, and his/her interactions with self and seeing the self from the other's perspective are integrated into field experience and written accounts (Hammersley & Atkinson, 1983; Rosenberg, 1990). We are interested in the taken-for-granted and often unexplored aspects of research such as the emotion work necessary to getting a study under way and the messy research realities that go undocumented, undiscussed and undisclosed; we argue that messy realities motivate us towards emotional reflexivity. Making our accounts and experiences available to others is the goal of this book. We hope to engage postgraduate researchers and supervisors in what we have learned by casting a reflexive eye on emotions in the field.

All the contributors to this book believe that emotions are inherent to knowledge production during the research process (Hochschild, 1983; Jaggar, 1989; Walkerdine, Lucey, & Melody, 2001; Holland, 2008); equally that credible research is as much about how you sample from your population as it is about how you situate yourself in the research (Neuman & Neumann, 2015). When planning and designing research, we may be unaware of our own emotional involvement in topics. In fact, we may with hindsight be blind to our own motivation in choosing certain topics (Neuman & Neumann, 2015; Pillow, 2003). Some sensitive research situations such as those involving end-of-life situations can be challenging. For example, personal and professional experiences of illness may come together, leading to heightened sensitivity within the research. These experiences are discussed in the chapters that follow.

In this book we argue for an emotional reflexivity. Our approach to using emotional reflexivity enables insight into ourselves and others. When we are aware of what we and our research participants are experiencing, this can lead to 'empathic insight' (Boden, Gibson, Owen, & Benson, 2016). It is impossible, we suggest, to understand the illness experience without trying to understand the emotional experience of an illness that is shared with us and observed by us, and such experiences require reflection and interpretation (Boden et al., 2016). Emotional reflexivity enables the impact of the research on the researcher and the participants to become visible rather than hidden and leads to rich insights as emotions motivate us to reflexivity. We have observed that the emotional impact of research is messy, challenging as well as rewarding. In this book we explore what doing emotional reflexivity consists of using the practical aspects of field research experienced by the contributors to the book.

Aims of the Book

In this book we have three aims:

- Explore how emotions motivate reflexivity in research practice
- Explore emotional involvement in the field
- Identify reflexive strategies which can be adopted through journaling, internal dialogues, peer support, clinical as well as academic supervision

Through the stories told by the contributors to this book, we unpack what emotional involvement in field research means for doing reflexivity. As reflexivity is a complex term with many interpretations, we define what this term means for each of us in each chapter. We expand the concept of emotional reflexivity as a pervasive element of reflexivity (Rosenberg, 1990), and an aspect of reflexivity which includes feelings (Boden et al., 2016). Using emotional reflexivity helps us to recognize our own emotions during fieldwork such as feelings of anger, injustices, embarrassment, sadness and numbness through observations of body language and our senses; in order to interpret these reflexively. In this book we draw on research carried out in highly sensitive settings including palliative care, adoption for people who are human immunodeficiency virus (HIV) positive, end-of-life care in Africa, couples and infertility, and young people who bully to explore the troubles and rewards experienced in the field.

All the contributing authors have a dual identity as researchers and health or social work professionals—Kit Tapson is a researcher and counsellor with young people; Tam Chipawe Cane is a social worker and researcher; Helen Allan, Anne Arber and Sarah Li are social scientists and trained nurses; Nicola Ayers as well as being a trained nurse has worked with refugees in Yemen and Ginny Mounce is a researcher and midwife. Doing research in sensitive settings involving loss, grief and social exclusion can be burdensome to the researcher. We found that in writing this book, the researchers did not always have the support they needed during fieldwork; in fact, they sometimes felt that their emotional involvement in the research was not relevant to academic supervision and that it was a private matter to find their own resources for support. Being aware of the emotional impact of research is important as researchers are human beings, and seeing and hearing devastating stories can be unsettling and upsetting.

Research Relationships and Emotions

The difficulty of being alive to emotions in the field and being at risk from those emotions is well described in work by Pillow (2003), Ramsay (1996) and Down, Garrety, and Badham (2006). The risks can be intensified if the field is gendered (Bloor, Fincham, & Sampson, 2007) or if the "amount of emotion work [the researcher does] in order not to show emotions" is burdensome (Down et al., 2006 cited by Holland, 2008, p. 19). All of the contributing chapters in this book illustrate how "the face-to-face proximity of the researchers to people whose stories are heavy with sorrow, loss, disappointment, anger and grief coupled with inequalities and social injustice make it easy to understand that there will be an emotional cost to undertaking these kinds of studies" (Bloor et al., 2007, p. 25).

A concern with the etic/emic relationships is central to all qualitative and quantitative research; that is, the comparisons between the outsider (researcher) and insider (native) worldviews and the theoretical explanations which derive from them (Robertson & Boyle, 1984). However, Bell (1993) argues that etic/emic positions become increasingly blurred as gender and ethnicity shape fieldwork. At times the researcher is no longer the outsider but may sometimes share in the experiences that they are researching.[1] The blurring that can occur between outsider and insider perspectives is both creative and dynamic, and will be discussed in several of the chapters. For example, the emotional fall out from experiencing rejection when wishing to be an insider (Chap. 2), feeling an insider and the tension this can engender when emotions are hidden (Chap. 3), insider and outsider identities and how they are managed between professional and the personal (Chaps. 4, 5, 7), managing strong emotions and flexing in action (Chap. 6) and blurring of boundaries between researcher and research participants (Chap. 8). Going native was seen as a real risk for ethnographers in the past because it meant empathizing with the 'natives' and becoming subjectively involved with them, which resulted (it was feared) in an inability to retain an objective, realist stance. Nowadays our fieldwork relationships are more reciprocal formed by both ourselves and our participants. Participants are also active in creating our field relationships (Bell, 1993; Hubbard, Backett-Milburn, & Kemmer, 2010; Neuman & Neumann, 2015; Vinten, 1994). Who we are and how we are in the field, our relationships in the field are important dimensions of fieldwork and the capacity for emotional reflexivity.

In qualitative fieldwork in health and social care settings, the researcher acknowledges that they themselves are grounded in a particular theoretical framework (Allen, 2004; Allan, 2011). Finken (2000) says that ethnography has three attributes: participant observation, interviews and documentary analysis, which are theoretically driven and applied using a particular philosophical stance. However, the attributes identified by Finken (2000) also overlap with other theoretically informed approaches such as grounded theory, case study research as well as phenomenological approaches and intervention studies. Our contributors have used a range of methodological approaches to fieldwork.

Interviews have become one of the most common methods of collecting data in health and social care settings, leading to observations of the 'interview society' where interviews are seen as a way of making sense of a life and of an illness (Atkinson & Silverman, 1997). Alongside this, we are also thought to be living in the 'observation society' where observing and being observed are features of Western society through access to mobile technology and webcams (Gobo & Marciniak, 2016). The contributors to this book use interviews and observations as a part of fieldwork. There are times in the book when researchers describe how they wished to close down the conversation when an emotion was expressed because they felt uncomfortable exploring certain aspects of illness experiences. At other times they describe being able to contain the pain of listening and feeling to allow the participant to express their feeling, to sit with the pain and acknowledge it instead of seeing it as disruptive. Clearly this intense engagement with those suffering from serious health conditions calls for emotion work and reflexivity on the part of the researcher.

One consequence of being a practitioner researcher is that one doesn't leave the field as such. For example, one of the contributors to the book, is now working with the people she researched (Chap. 7). Williams (1990) writes about this and suggests that distinctions between being in the field (being there) and being out of the field (being here—back safely in academia) are to an extent false. The relationship between being there/in and here/out of the field is perhaps more accurately conceptualized as being on a continuum in a relationship *with* the field. Following Savage (2003), we suggest that the practitioner researcher moves between the different ways of being in the field in a dynamic way; in fact, multiple identities may be taken as well as given. The investment by the researcher in the practice setting can result in close relationships resulting in receptivity to changes in practice reminiscent of action research. Having an insider understanding of the practice context can result in rich descriptions, but on the other hand, insider understanding and knowledge may blind one to other interesting aspects of the field.

Emotions and Reflexivity

Underpinning our discussion of emotional reflexivity is the assumption that emotions, whether we are unconscious or conscious of them, shape our everyday life through their effect on our relationships with others and on our own internal psyche (Jacobs, 1999). As Jacobs (1999) suggests, psyche encompasses mind, self, emotions and spirit. By using the term *psyche*, we are deliberately drawing attention to the complexity of our internal, emotional lives which become even more complex when doing fieldwork where we are confronted with our own and *others'* emotions (Evans, Periera, & Parker, 2012). Each of the contributors has reflected on their own positioning in the field, their understanding, emotional experience of *self* and other through reflections from research diaries, journals and blogs.

It is possible that researchers through their experience of emotions, or ignoring emotions, can be negatively affected (Holland, 2007). It is difficult to know to what extent we should be emotionally involved with those we engage with in research. Many textbooks discuss emotional involvement as hindering research efforts; for example, leading one off track by a key informant for example and blurring the boundary between the participant and the researcher. Emotional expression by the participant could also potentially harm the researcher who may not have adequate support and have to grapple with strong emotions engendered by the research on their own. However, telling stories about difficult illness experiences and having space to tell one's story for the first time (Hughes & Arber, 2008) can be liberating and enables participants to have a voice about suffering and loss that could otherwise go unheard. Likewise, the emotions experienced by the researcher do not have to harm the research. Although emotions may be processed by writing about them, we have found in this book that they can be neglected with the researcher left to process them alone. Atunement to feelings may exist already as part of the individual researcher's practice and skills. This atunement can be encouraged through use of some of the strategies described in this book that motivate to emotional reflexivity. Ways to express emotions and feel comfortable with this expression can be developed with supervisory and institutional support and modelling by supervisors.

Overview of Chapters

Chapter 2 identifies key features of reflexivity from the literature and then explores the natural history of a Ph.D. study using an ethnomethodological gaze. The emotional impact of setting out on the research journey is explored and troubled moments are revealed throughout the journey towards a Ph.D.

Chapter 3 discusses the role of observation and interviews in illuminating hidden emotions in the fertility clinic in both participants and the observer. Moments when the personal and professional collide which motivate towards a reflexivity of emotions are described.

Chapter 4 discusses the dual identity of the researcher as a practitioner and how that was handled and reflected on. Reputation became a key construct in the research and developed from a reflexivity of the dual role and how that dual role impacted on insider identity and reputation in research conducted in hospice and palliative care.

Chapter 5 discusses the challenges associated with HIV-related infertility and participants' experiences of seeking parenthood. Tensions between the researcher position, recruitment of participants to the research, ethical challenges and confidentiality erupted in unexpected ways and resulted in an emotional fallout.

Chapter 6 identifies the challenges of being a counsellor and researcher when researching marginalized groups of young people who are difficult to reach. The emotional and the psychological safety of both researcher and participants are discussed in relation to emotion work and emotion management.

Chapter 7 explores the challenges when conducting fieldwork in another culture. Reflexive practices helped towards an understanding that the researcher was neither neutral nor passive. Balancing the insider and outsider identity in the research was the motivation to reflexivity.

Chapter 8 explores the tensions inherent in sustained involvement with research participants over time where the researcher becomes close to participants. The challenges regarding researcher identity and boundaries in a setting where the researcher is known are reflected upon.

Chapter 9 brings together the key implications for emotional reflexivity including researcher support strategies, training for academic supervisors, the importance of clinical supervision and strategies to achieve emotional reflexivity during the natural history of the research.

Notes

1. See Williams (1990) on this point.

References

Allan, H. T. (2011). Using psycho-dynamic small group work in nurse education: Closing the theory-practice gap? *Nurse Education Today, 31*(5), 521–524.

Allen, D. (2004). Ethnomethodological insights into insider-outsider relationships. *Nursing Inquiry, 11*(1), 14–24.

Atkinson, P., & Silverman, D. (1997). Kindera's immortality: The interview society and the invention of the self. *Qualitative Inquiry, 3*, 304–325.

Bell, D. (1993). Introduction 1, the context. In D. Bell, P. Caplan, & J. W. Karim (Eds.), *Gendered fields, women, men and ethnography* (pp. 1–18). London: Routledge.

Bloor, M., Fincham, B., & Sampson, H. (2007). *Commissioned inquiry into the risk to well-being of researchers in qualitative research.* Cardiff: Qaultiti (NCRM).

Boden, Z. V. R., Gibson, S., Owen, G. J., & Benson, O. (2016). Feelings and intersubjectivity in qualitative research. *Qualitative Health Research, 26*(8), 1078–1090.

Cain, C. (2012). Emotions and the research interview: What hospice workers can teach us. *Health Sociology Review, 21*(4), 396–405.

Down, S., Garrety, K., & Badham, R. (2006). Fear and loathing in the field: Emotional dissonance and identity work in ethnographic research. *Management, 9*(3), 87–107.

Evans, A., Periera, D., & Parker, J. (2012). Categorising the nurse-researcher during fieldwork: 'One of us' or 'one of them'? *Journal of Research in Nursing, 18*(8), 707–717.

Finken, S. (2000). *Bringing ethnography home, reflections upon a style of enquiry.* Retrieved March 1, 2016, from http://citeseerx.ist.psu.edu/viewdoc/download?doi=10.1.1.25.9078&rep=rep1&type=pdf

Finlay, L. (2002). Negotiating the swamp: The opportunity and challenge of reflexivity in research practice. *Qualitative Research, 2*(2), 209–230.

Gobo, G., & Marciniak, L. T. (2016). What is ethnography? In D. Silverman (Ed.), *Qualitative research* (pp. 103–120). London: Sage.

Hammersley, M. (1992). On feminist methodology. *Sociology, 26*(2), 187–206.

Hammersley, M., & Atkinson, P. (1983). *Ethnography: Principles in practice.* London: Routledge.

Hochschild, A. (1983). *The managed heart: The commercialisation of human feeling.* Berkley, CA: University of California Press.

Holland, J. (2007). Emotions and research. *International Journal of Social Research Methodology, 10*(3), 195–209.

Holland, J. (2008). Emotions and research: Some general and personal thoughts. In S. Weller & C. Caballero (Eds.), *Up close and personal: Relationships and emotions within and through research* (pp. 11–12). Families & Social Capital Research Group Working Paper No. 25, South Bank University, London. Retrieved from https://www.lsbu.ac.uk/__.../up-close-personal-relationships-emotions-families-researc...

Hubbard, G., Backett-Milburn, K., & Kemmer, D. (2010). Working with emotions: Issues for the researcher in fieldwork and teamwork. *International Journal of Social Research Methodology, 4*, 119–137.

Hughes, N., & Arber, A. (2008). The lived experience of patients with pleural mesothelioma. *International Journal of Palliative Nursing, 14*, 66–71.

Jacobs, M. (1999). *Psychodynamic counselling in action* (2nd ed.). London: Sage Publications.

Jaggar, A. (1989). Love and knowledge: Emotion in feminist epistemology. In S. Bordo & A. Jaggar (Eds.), *Gender/body/knowledge: Feminist reconstructions of being and knowing*. New Brunswick; London: Rutgers University Press.

Neuman, C. B., & Neumann, I. B. (2015). Uses of the self: Two ways of thinking about scholarly situatedness and method. *Millennium, Journal of International Studies, 43*(3), 798–819.

Pillow, W. S. (2003). Confession, catharsis or sure? Rethinking the uses of reflexivity as methodological power in qualitative research. *Qualitative Studies in Education, 16*(2), 175–196.

Ramsay, K. (1996). Emotional labour and qualitative research: How I learned not to laugh or cry in the field. In E. S. Lyon & J. Busfield (Eds.), *Methodological imaginations* (pp. 131–1460). Basingstoke: Macmillan.

Robertson, M., & Boyle, J. (1984). Ethnography: Contributions to nursing research. *Journal of Advanced Nursing, 9*(1), 43–49.

Rosenberg, M. (1990). Reflexivity and emotions. *Social Psychology Quarterly, 53*(1), 3–12.

Savage, J. (2003). Participative observation. In J. Latimer (Ed.), *Advanced qualitative research for nursing* (pp. 53–76). Oxford: Blackwell Science Ltd.

Seale, C. (1999). *The quality of qualitative research*. London: Sage.

Vinten, G. (1994). Participant observation: A model for organisational investigation? *Journal of Managerial Psychology, 9*(2), 30–38.

Walkerdine, V., Lucey, H., & Melody, J. (2001). *Growing up girl: Psychosocial explorations of gender and class*. Basingstoke: Palgrave.

Williams, A. (1990). *Reflections on the making of an ethnographic text*. Studies in Sexual Politics, No. 29. Manchester: Manchester University Press.

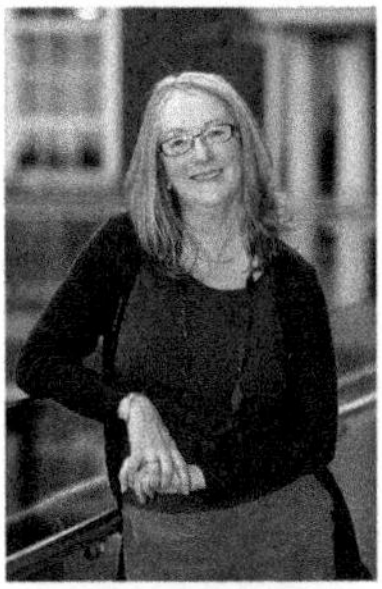

Helen T. Allan is Professor in Nursing at the Centre for Critical Research in Nursing & Midwifery, Middlesex University, London, UK. Helen was awarded her Ph.D. in 2000 from the Royal College of Nursing Institute/University of Manchester. Helen has supervised Ph.D. and clinical doctorates since 2002.

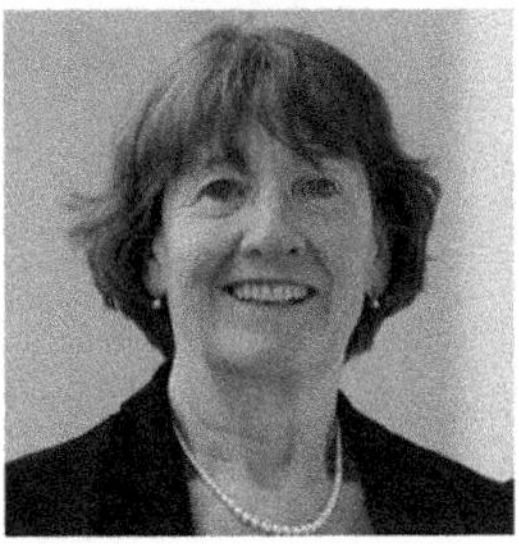

Anne Arber is Senior Lecturer in Cancer and Palliative Care, School of Health Sciences, University of Surrey, Guildford, Surrey, UK. Anne was awarded her Ph.D. in 2004 from Goldsmiths, University of London, UK. Anne conducts research in cancer and palliative care. She has supervised Ph.D. and clinical doctorate students since 2004.

2

The Natural History of a Doctoral Research Study: The Role of a Research Diary and Reflexivity

Sarah Li

Introduction

The aim of this chapter is to make a strong case for the role of a research diary as a site for reflexivity. I will describe what reflexivity looks like in practice, demonstrate how I 'do' reflexivity and the strategies I used to do it in my PhD. I will produce a model of reflexivity in practice. Alongside this, critical moments documented in my research diary, where moments of emotional reflexivity occurred, will be made visible. I start by discussing what I've called the natural history of my doctoral research.

It has been suggested that topics for a natural history of research could include the personal context, the micro-analysis of social interaction, reasons for the research design developing through trial and error and methodological lessons that were learned. The data in this chapter are drawn from extracts from my research diary which I kept during my doctoral research journey and involve 65 diary entries from September 1999 to October 2002 (Li, 2001, 2002a, 2002b, 2003). Additional materials

S. Li (✉)
St George's, University of London, London, UK

H.T. Allan, A. Arber (eds.), *Emotions and reflexivity in Health and Social Care Field Research*, https://doi.org/10.1007/978-3-319-65503-1_2

analysed in the course of this project, some of which are referred to in this chapter, include 17 written records of the supervision reports made by the supervisor and agreed by me as the student, 19 taped tutorials, five annual progress reports written by me for years 2, 3 and 5, and my field notes. The records provided physical evidence of actions taken (Borg, 2001) and my progress and achievements during the PhD. They enhance the quality and credibility of my accounts. The grounded theory approach was adopted and conversational analysis (Garfinkel, 1967, 1992) was used to explicate the seen but unnoticed features of reflexivity. I called this analytic tool the 'ethnomethodological gaze'. Ethnomethology is the study of folk practices (Garfinkel, 1967), and gaze, the power of the eye (Foucault, 1963). My approach served as an added eye (Beck, Giddens, et al. 1994) to uncover critical moments of reflexivity. However, it is beyond the scope of this chapter to discuss details of my methodologies here. I refer the readers to my published work elsewhere (Li, 2005; Li & Seale, 2007a, 2007b, 2007c, 2008).

My research diary was longitudinal and chronological; it spanned six years (I studied part time) and was recorded at different stages of the doctoral experience (Li, 2002a, 2002b). It documents my thinking, my interest and emotional investment, dilemmas, troubles, setbacks and challenges. It documents how these processes and events shaped my behaviour and my future actions (Borg, 2001; Engin, 2011). Through a close reading of my diary, critical moments of reflexivity and emotional reactions are located. In this chapter, I categorize critical moments into practical, theoretical, analytical, emotional and personal in the practice of reflexivity.

At the start of my doctoral journey, I found little consensus in the way the concept of reflexivity was described in the research literature. The concept itself was ambiguously defined (Nadin & Cassell, 2006); even more confusingly, Beck et al. (1994) argued that reflection was conceptually distinct from reflexivity. Beck et al. (1994) understand reflection as social knowledge or seeing things with an 'added eye' (p. 175). Reflexivity was understood as 'unintentional or unseen self-dissolution' (p. 175), 'self-endangerment' (p. 176), a sense of 'self-application', 'self-criticism' or 'self-modification' (p. 179). They defined reflexivity as a systematic reflection on the 'unconscious presuppositions' categories of our knowledge (p. 176). Yet they did not expand on just what these presuppositions meant in practical terms. I now discuss current debates around reflexivity drawing on work published since my PhD.

Being Reflexive

Finlay (2002) suggest that the practice of reflexivity involves reflection, thinking and self-dialogue, culminating in exciting discoveries about an intense interest, conflicting positions and concerns that call out to the researcher to pursue and explore. And Alvesson and Skoldberg (2009) consider reflexivity as an action of reflection, which includes:

> The attention paid to the way different kinds of linguistic, social, political and theoretical elements are woven together in the process of knowledge development, during which empirical material is constructed, interpreted and written… (Alvesson & Skoldberg, 2009, p. 9).

Alvesson and Skoldberg (2009) present reflexivity as a way of seeing and understanding what happens at regular intervals in the research process. Reflexivity is socially constructed, constantly shaped by the contexts and culture in which researchers work (May & Perry, 2010). Alvesson and Skoldberg (2009) present three forms of reflexivity: self-reflexivity, domain reflexivity and collaborative reflexivity (p. 3). Domain reflexivity (p. 5) involves more than one researcher working together in terms of collecting and interpreting data, comparing notes and interpretations. Collaborative reflexivity involves sharing information, feedback and reflecting on practice. For Alvesson and Skoldberg (2009), self-reflexivity refers to the act of reflecting on how a researcher's own embedded influence might shape the research outcomes during fieldwork. For example, Arber (2006) found that the juxtaposition of her dual role as an academic researcher and practitioner created extraordinary interactional difficulties and dilemmas. She found that the acceptance of her roles by participants as an insider and outsider was contingent upon the cultural context she was in. She managed this difficulty by shifting her position from going native, avoiding, withdrawing and pulling back to the position of peacemaker, who smoothed and negotiated.

Finlay (2002) defined reflexivity as 'introspection' (p. 213) and 'social critique' (p. 220). Introspection refers to an internal search for meaning through an examination of one's own experience and personal meanings. Social critique refers to the power dynamic between researcher and the researched, and how this power relationship is collaboratively managed in the research process. This is an example of what Alvesson and Skoldberg (2009) call 'collaborative reflexivity' (p. 3). They suggest that we need to recognize the co-existence of two distinct types of expertise possessed by academic researchers whom the authors called 'the theoria' (p. 3), and the professional expertise possessed by the practitioners whom they called the 'praxia' (p. 3). The co-existence of two distinct forms of expertise helps promote mutual improvements and anchors the relevance of empirical research.

All social relationships are affected by interpersonal dynamics in everyday social encounters (Singnal & Jeffrey, 2008). Buscatto (2016) cautions us to strike a balance between 'maintaining distance' and 'remaining detached' (p. 140). For Buscatto, reflexivity involves constant flexibility and adaptability in order to accommodate changes as they arise in the course of our research journey. Reflexivity offers a voyage of adventure, an emotional experience in a constant process of watchfulness (watching oneself) and thoughtfulness (Singnal & Jeffrey, 2008).

Engward and Davis (2015), drawing from case examples, found that practicing reflexivity involves a process of 'critical self-reflection on one's bias, theoretical predispositions and preferences' (p. 1532). Critical self-reflection involves the activities of questioning (for example, assumptions and preconceived ideas), checking and re-checking (their own understanding of what was happening), including or excluding bits that were not relevant (for example, in sampling and data analysis). Such activities help to tidy up the messy reality of the research process, and enable researchers to make rational decisions in order to move on. Malaurent and Avison (2017) describe reflexivity as a complex process of 'thinking and experience' or 'interpretation of interpretation' (p. 1). Hertz (1997, p. viii) suggests practicing reflexivity involves 'an ongoing conversation about the experience whilst simultaneously living in the moment'. It entails constant self-assessment of knowledge and ways of doing it, a continuous process of questioning and evaluating in practice. This self-assessment results in the production of a rigorous research outcome. Nadin and Cassell (2006) suggest that reflexivity involves 'thinking about our own thinking' (p. 209). Enosh (2016, p. 578) argues that reflexivity involved 'a deliberate awareness of thinking and acting on' and 'a constant movement of being in the phenomenon and stepping outside of it'. Enosh calls this process 'reflexivity and reactivity' (p. 578). It is suggested that the process of self-questioning about methodological, theoretical and practical issues should be practiced from the beginning to the end of the research (Silverman, 2010a).

In summary, the collective message from the literature seems to be that reflexivity is an important research device for the social construction of new knowledge and the production of competent research identities. The main strategy for doing reflexivity involves thinking, experiencing and acting to shape research outcomes. Strategies for acting on that thinking gleaned from the empirical literature include vetting and checking, watching, maintaining distancing and remaining detached, tidying and cleaning up, avoiding (Silverman, 2010b), withdrawing and pulling back, peace-making, smoothing and negotiating (Arber, 2006). In the next section, I will explore the role of research diary in reflexivity.

The Research Diary

There has been a growing interest in the role of the research diary in doing reflexivity, and how the diary is used for reflexivity in doctoral research (Borg, 2001; Arber, 2006; Nadin & Cassell, 2006; Potter, 2006; Rapley, 2007; Silverman, 2010b; Engin, 2011). The main consensus is that the research diary is a record of thoughts, emotions and discussions with self and others. It is an important site for the practice of reflexivity, as well as the production of new knowledge. A research diary used reflexively documents how a researcher develops from a novice to a competent and independent researcher. For example, Borg (2001, p. 161) concludes that the research diary provided 'instructive insight' into specific aspects of the research process. It played an important role in shaping his thinking. The activities of thinking Borg undertook led to significant discoveries which enabled him to move on and successfully complete his doctoral research. He used thinking and self-questioning as the main devices to get answers, clarify bias and assumptions. He dealt with anxiety (i.e. meeting deadlines) by using devices such as 'getting off', 'opening up' and 'bringing out' his pent-up emotions in his diary. He dealt with negative feedback and the dilemma of the final writing- up by using devices such as 'questioning and re-evaluating', 'stopping and returning to', 'getting rid of and moving on', and 'moving away and entering into' (a therapeutic relationship). These devices enabled him to make decisions about the structure of his thesis and what it would look like. His research diary provided physical evidence of his progress which motivated him and gave him a positive sense of 'achievement' (Borg, 2001, p. 171).

Nadin and Cassell (2006) provide another example of how reflexivity was practiced using a research diary in the context of the management of self. Nadin and Cassell (2006, p. 214), using the research diary, developed the following strategies in the early stages of data analysis. These were: 'thinking ahead and reflecting back', 'engaging with and remaining detached', and 'reading and wider reading'. Such strategies resulted in reducing data and establishing the link between theory and method. Nadin dealt with her emotions and anger arising from fieldwork by 'letting go and opening up', 'questioning', 'visiting and re-visiting' what she had done. She realized that anger may impact upon the interpretation of the transcript. So for her, the research diary was a useful substitute when there was 'no-one to have a conversation with' (p. 214). This also demonstrates the importance of emotions experienced during fieldwork and the diary as a strategy for emptying out strong emotion.

Silverman (2010c) presented personal stories of three of his former Doctoral students, M, S, and Sn, who kept research diaries throughout their PhDs. The diaries documented how their initial ideas emerged and changed in response to the factors that arose during their doctoral research journey. They documented their personal impact on their fieldwork, decisions they made about methods of data collection, analytical approach and the lessons learned. For example, M found that the emerging topics she thought important were not treated as relevant by her participants. This insight prompted her to question her own assumptions and bias, and then took a 'step back' to take a 'closer look' at the phenomenon under investigation. A series of activities followed, which involved 'reading and re-reading' her transcripts for a detailed fine-grained analysis. S and Sn dealt with the messy reality of data analysis by using the strategies of 'listening/re-listening' to audio recordings; 'examining', 'reading and re-reading' their field notes; 'defining/re-defining' categories; 'rejecting', 'moving away', 'narrowing down', 'searching for' and 'taking on' new findings (Silverman, 2010c, p. 41). These activities are similar to Engin's (2011) reflexive activities, the result of thinking processes and 'noticings' (p. 302). The writing entailed in keeping a research diary establishes the importance of writing as thinking (Rapley, 2007). Rapley said: 'writing is thinking, you may think you have a clear idea, but it is only when you write it down that you can be certain that you do' (p. 25). Thus, the articulation of thoughts and feelings documented in the students' research diaries becomes the catalyst for change in beliefs and practice through narratives and self-dialogue and the ability to move on (Engin, 2011).

In my doctoral thesis (Li, 2002a, 2002b), I investigated how palliative care nurses enact psychosocial care in their natural settings (two hospices and one general hospital), with reference to their *talk*. The aim of the thesis was to relate the doing of psychosocial care to broader notions of nursing as a form of emotional labour. The thesis offered an ethnomethodological-ethnographic perspective on psychosocial care and advanced a theory that 'symbiotic niceness' was co-produced and co-performed in interaction by participants. This process of interactional co-production of niceness (Li, 2002a, 2002b) served as a means of managing relations between palliative care nurses and dying patients. At the first seminar for first year Doctoral students at Goldsmith's Sociology department, David Silverman emphasized the importance of keeping a research diary to keep track of how researchers' ideas change during the research process, which is discussed next.

Reflexivity in Practice: My Story

I start with an early diary entry to illustrate feelings of loss and grief reactions, which I experienced at the beginning of my story:

> Feeling a bit bereft of Goldsmith's atmosphere after a year's break on completion of my MA sociology. My children have 'flown' the nest. Experiencing the 'empty nest syndrome'. Thinking about doing a PhD. My topic: what

does it mean to give psychosocial care in care of the terminally ill/dying. (Research Diary Li, 2001)

This diary entry was triggered by three critical moments of reflexivity through thinking, self-questioning and emotional experience (Malaurent & Avison, 2017; Nadin & Cassell, 2006). The first moment occurred when I suffered a dreadful empty nest feeling after completing a Master degree in Sociology. I was working full time as a Senior Lecturer at Kingston University at the time. My children had left home and I was worried about losing my academic ability and credibility. I felt I needed to step out of that empty feeling mood and move on! I wanted to go back to Goldsmith's College! The second moment was when my father became terminally ill with cancer in Hong Kong. I had to return home to Hong Kong at his request. He was admitted into an expensive private hospital. However, in the two weeks I was there, I noticed that it was my mother who cared for my father. The nurses were wafting in and out of my father's room, just to give medications and dress the wounds, albeit with the occasional 'hello' in between. There was very little interaction between the nurses and my father. I felt that the nurses had abandoned care to my mother. A question came to my mind: 'Aren't they supposed to be giving their patients holistic care that was supposed to be the conventional wisdom in the care of the terminally ill?' (Saunders & Baines, 1983). The issue which concerned me was the relation between what was taught and approved within terminal care and what nurses actually did (Li, 2002a, 2002b).

The third moment occurred when I conducted an observational study in an elderly care ward in a small general hospital in South London (Li, 1985). I observed that nurses were trying to straighten up an imminently dying woman's limbs and head from a semi-prone position (Li, 2002a, 2002b). This incident reminded me of a form of premature social death imposed on the living bodies of dying patients (Sudnow, 1967). I felt and experienced the vulnerability and loneliness of this dying patient. I became interested in how 'psychosocial care' was practiced in palliative care settings. Thus, reflexivity in theses instance of diary entries led to a change a transition of role from a professional role (as a Senior Lecturer) to the role of a PhD research student. Feelings and experiencing loss, thinking, noticing, observing, self-questioning, remembering, reminding were motivations for reflexivity in these three moments. 'Looking back' and 'going back', 'stepping out and moving on' were my strategies for acting on these experiences. The outcome of these activities led to my first turning point, which was to register for a PhD in Sociology, and secure my choice of a supervisor in CS, as my diary entries testified below:

> Wanted CS to be my supervisor as he has expertise in my field of interest, as well as research methodologies. That is what I needed. Didn't want anybody else. Tested other waters, didn't like them. (Research Diary Li, 2001)

> Met with CS. He agreed. Yippee! (Research diary Li, 2001)

The next stage of reflexivity was my entry into the field, by *getting in*:

> What am I going to do? I don't know anybody! Where do I start? God I am so shy. Talking to 'strangers' is not a hobby of mine! (Research Diary Li, 2001)

The diary entry above revealed a critical moment of self-questioning, anxiety and worries about beginning. I began negotiating access to palliative care settings for my fieldwork. The implication these questions posed was about dealing with the messy reality of data collection in unfamiliar settings. I felt shy with strangers, who could potentially be my gatekeepers. I always felt uncomfortable talking to people I did not know. Worrying about it led to decisions about the number of research settings I needed. Initially I thought of looking at palliative care units in general hospitals in Central London, as well as in my own locality where I worked. However I had to narrow down the choice of settings in order for my study to be workable and achievable (Silverman, 2010a), as my diary entry testified below:

> Worried about not getting access from some settings, I decided to look at several settings for safe-keeping. Eventually, I might have to narrow down my fieldwork as I might end up with too much data. (Research Diary Li, 2001)

Silverman (2010c) advises us to draw upon our own contacts and experience as far as possible. My worries flagged up in this critical moment, prompted me to talk and seek advice from my colleague (AA) who had contacts in three palliative care settings. She suggested that I used the more user-friendly (informal) approach (telephoning) to gently ease myself into each of these settings, as the entry below testified:

> Talked to my colleague AA…She suggested trying to make contact by phone first. A written request would be too formal. May scare people off… so they are the real gate-keepers I thought. (Research Diary Li, 2001)

Before I met senior managers, doctors, social workers and palliative care nurses, I thought carefully about how to make them like me and accept me: how would I relate to members in the field? As Coffey (1999) reminds us, fieldwork is dependent on making relationships with people in a personal way. I made a conscious decision to introduce myself as a Registered Nurse first and then as a Senior Lecturer. Like (Arber, 2006), I thought if I presented myself as one of them, that is to say, one who held approved nursing qualification as they did, I felt it would give me credibility and win trust, as my diary entry below testified (H is the senior manager):

> Gosh, what a crowd! Mrs. H said as soon as I got the go ahead, I could sit in on their meetings and start my observation! I wondered: would these lovely people be so eager to support me if I were not 'one of them', so to speak? (Research Diary Li, 2001)

However, to my utter embarrassment, I discovered that getting in as an insider was not enough. I still had to present myself as a credible person with a credible CV, as my diary entry testified below:

> Made contact with hospice number three, a well- established hospice. Asked for a covering letter, my protocol, a supporting statement from Clive and my CV! What on earth are they looking for? What else do they want from me, my bank statement? (Research Diary Li, 2001)

I was asked to 'tone down' my language in one of my letters to a Senior Manager and 'take a step back'; causing offence in interaction broke all the rules necessary for smooth social interaction (Goffman, 1976a, 1976b). I had hit a 'controlled zone' and had to make a U-turn! Otherwise I could have sabotaged my study. This was a wake-up call for me as my diary entry below testified:

> Disaster! Phone from Mrs. H. (hospital 2). She was not pleased with my letter to Dr. M. Said I needed to tone it down a bit. Was I being too pushy? A bit scary of her. Asked me to take a step back! I offered to amend the letter. She said no need. She would speak to the doctor. Felt a bit slighted by this. H reiterated her full support for me. Felt reassured. (Research Diary Li, 2001)

I learned then that I was watched *as I watched others* (Singnal & Jeffrey, 2008). I had to watch my step from this point onwards and pay attention to language (Alvesson & Skoldberg, 2009), as this was important in building a good relationships with gatekeepers. This discovery marked a second turning point where reflexivity (questioning, thinking) and reactivity (acting on that thinking) as suggested by Enosh (2016) flagged up critical issues related to how I interacted with participants. I learned to deal with these interactional difficulties by 'easing in, taking a step back, narrowing down, talking and seeking advice, toning down and amending'. In this instance, as my entry above testified, by performing my U-turn and learning through reflexivity, I had gained initial acceptance and 'full support'. I was given the green light to start field observation, as my diary entries testified below:

> Permission granted by Mrs. H to start phase one of my project: observation. (Research Diary Li, 2001)

> Met B and new palliative care nurse AJ at hospital one. They were very happy for me to start. They would identify patients of terminal care for me. (Research Diary Li, 2001)

The next stage was *getting along and staying in*, which referred to a period during which I began my data collection in the first research setting. I was allowed to sit in on the hand-over meetings between two shifts of nurses and listen to the most intimate details of dying patients. I thought I was accepted as an insider. I was wrong. I thought that once I had gained permission from the research ethics committee to use an audio recorder, I took it for granted that I had a passport for everything else. In my naivety as a novice researcher, I was unprepared for many unseen and unexpected roadblocks on the roads, as my diary entry below revealed:

> Went to H2 setting to audio-record nurses' hand-over. L (nurse) said not to use the audio-recorder as she said: 'it is confidential'. Felt totally downhearted. Only spent an hour there. (Research Diary Li, 2001)

I felt I had been sent back into the world of an outsider. This sudden realization prompted me to take a step back, abandon my taken-for-granted attitude and adopt a flexible position in which I switched between an insider role and an outsider role to suit the situation as it arose. I learned that I had to constantly negotiate and renegotiate consent from my participants. I realized I had to work at getting along and staying in (Kirk & Miller, 1986). I would be reminded of my outsider status time and time again and I had to remind myself that I was only a guest after all. Reflexivity in this instance gave me opportunities to rethink my attitude, abandon any taken-for-granted assumptions so I could get along and stay in. This realization prompted me to discuss this problem of recording with my ally (D) in the field. His response (below) shows, I had hit a dead end. Although there were utterances of delay and hesitation (oh...yes...um…), perhaps as he struggled to disagree with me, nevertheless, the answer to my enquiry was 'no':

> I discussed with D (a palliative care nurse) about the problem of keeping up with nurses' talking and writing at the same time. I could not keep up with the speed of their talk. I said to him: 'I don't know what is the best way' as I hinted that it would be so much easier if I could use the audio-recorder. He looked at me: 'oh………yes……….yes…….um…….yes'. I took this response as a no-goer. (Research Diary Li, 2001)

Another difficult moment came during this phase when I felt I was 'cold-shouldered' by several of the palliative care nurses in this setting. I felt I was repeatedly treated as an unwanted outsider. The following entries in my research diary recorded this observation:

> Felt being ostracized by staff there. R (nurse) was nice. Sensed there was conflict of some sort amongst the staff there. The tension in the main office was evident when Dr. was there! I felt utterly rejected. No cups of tea. I was on my own wandering just outside the office. K (nurse) ignored me till I forced myself to say 'hello' to her. L then said: 'you have to accept what you see here' when I asked her if it was alright for me to sit in the office. What did she mean by that? I don't want to come back to this hospice to collect anymore data. Must talk to C (my supervisor) and my friend AA about this. I'd better latch onto D as he seemed nice also. (Research Diary Li, 2001)

This feeling of ostracism happened again with L, another palliative care nurse:

> I saw L in the car park to the hospice. She looked at me. I turned to greet her but she walked quickly up the steps away from me! Research Diary (Li, 2001)

> After the hand-over, they carried on chatting without registering me there. I felt awkward after 10 minutes writing. (Research Diary Li, 2001)

Clearly, my status as a nurse did not dissolve the distance between me and these nurses in these settings (Arber, 2006; Li, 2002a, 2002b). I was upset at what I thought was a coldness towards me. I thought all nurses would be welcoming. I wanted to leave the field. I felt utterly lost and rejected. My self-question prompted me to ask for help from my supervisor C and my friend AA, as my diary entry below testified:

> Must talk to C and my friend AA about this. (Research Diary Li, 2001)

The extract below was evident of the action I took. It was a record of supervision written by my supervisor to me. The 'we' below referred to my supervisor and I:

> We also discussed her experiences of fieldwork in hospice 2. Not a very friendly experience at this hospice, but potentially interesting setting to compare with the hospital and hospice 1. (Supervision Record)

My supervisor helped me to understand that what had happened could be interesting despite the fact I felt emotionally dejected. The implication from my experience was that my role as an outsider researcher might have increased their anxiety and suspicion that I was there to judge them (Hammersley & Atkinson, 1983). Like Arber (2006), I needed to tread the delicate boundary between insider and outsider carefully. I managed this awkward situation by becoming my own gatekeeper. I called this action 'self-censoring' through observation of the self. Evidence of this self-censorship is evident in my diary entries below (D and K are palliative care nurses):

> I wished I could go nearer the patients. Somehow I felt I did not have the liberty. The nurses all disappeared from the bedrooms. I took a quick peep but that was all. I am not getting anywhere. I think I might have to re-negotiate with D for more freedom. (Research Diary Li, 2001)

> K was talking about a patient in general who had apparently drove her to pieces. I did not write down what she said as I could read from her eyes that she did not want me to, so I didn't. (Research Diary Li, 2002a)

I was feeling daunted and unsure about how far I should go with my observations. I was also now recognizing emotions in the staff that meant I censored what I was writing down. I continued by stepping back and taking stock of what had happened, checking and re-checking my demeanour. I tried to maintain a nice front (Goffman, 1976a, 1976b), be courteous, friendly but not overtly friendly, and keep my counsel (Silverman, 2010b). I also offered to show my field notes to these two nurses because I wanted them to trust me. An entry in my research diary testified to this:

> I said: 'oh, you can read what I've just written. I am only interested in the words or language you used to describe your patients' conditions. (Research Diary Li, 2002a)

I reciprocated nurses' friendliness by offering my help (making tea for them). I maintained a polite demeanour (Goffman, 1967) by constantly seeking agreement through the process of negotiation and re-negotiation. I developed an acute sense of awareness which I called 'learned intuitiveness' (Li, 2002a, 2002b). This involved constantly reflecting on my field experiences in order to detect the slightest hint when I should politely withdraw my presence at critical moments. I also learned to pick up cues from nurses' non-verbal signs. My field note below would testify this: P is the patient, 'I' is (SL), both N1 (Nurse 1) and N2 (Nurse 2) are palliative care nurses:

> N1 came in to ask N2 to help her with P in Room 7. N2 went with N1 straight away. I followed them. P was on his bed. I could see his dressing but I decided not to go in as he has a lot of problems and he appeared to be in pain. I felt I did not want to intrude. (Field notes)

The outcome was that nurses were much more welcoming and they gave me complete access to the field. This opening-up is reflected in the supervision notes and diary extract below:

> S (SL) has collected a considerable body of data, having established good working relations in her field settings in the past year or two (Supervision Report)

> 'Felt much more welcomed by the nurses there especially K. I've come to like her as she is a straight talker. S sent me to the kitchen to make tea for myself and if I wanted to make tea for the day and night staff as well. I was so pleased to be able to do something for them once in return!' (Research diary Li, 2002a)

> 'Been to the hospice (2). Staff very friendly and welcoming. Much more at ease with me.' (Research Diary Li, 2002a)

As can be seen from the extracts above, being reflexive was prompted by critical moments in my relations with participants in the field. Being reflexive meant constantly taking a step back and taking stock, checking and re-checking, reciprocating, self-censoring and watching others. Reflexive practice led ultimately to a successful outcome as I had gained the nurses' trust. I had become an insider! I moved freely around the settings with guardedness and absolute respect. The act of self-censoring enabled me to stay in the field.

The next troubled moment arose when I was told in a joking manner not to record the nurses' conversations. This request was done not in a serious way (Li, 2002a, 2002b) as it was accompanied by laughter. G and L are palliative care nurses in the extract below:

> When I asked for the night staff's name, G said 'oh, you are going to write about me and incriminate me now (laughter).' (Research Diary Li, 2002a)

> At one point, L was joking about a patient. She turned to me and said: 'oh, don't write that down'. I said: 'oh no'. So I stopped writing. Everybody laughed when she said that. (Research Diary Li, 2002a)

Re-reading the above two diary entries outside the field stirred up a dilemma I faced, which I did not know how to deal with. To me as a researcher, the forbidden data were significant because they represented a part of reality that nurses did not want to reveal. This episode contradicted my thesis of 'symbiotic niceness' and became my deviant case in the thesis (Li, 2002a, 2002b). I named these data 'censored talk' (Li, 2002a, 2002b, p. 279). By 'censored talk' I meant parts of talk which were 'edited out' from the parts that were 'edited in' or 'approved'. I was specifically asked not to record this instance of talk. The talk was 'censored' by nurses when they appeared to be very critical of their patients in one setting. I discussed this issue with my supervisor, as the tutorial testified (CS is the supervisor, S is SL):

> CS: 'one question is erm … maybe all this niceness..is pretty untypical[?] [T]he way the nurses usually behave when a researcher is (around). (S: oh right) What would you say to that?
>
> S: … I would say that what I'm proposing is staged niceness..and that there is no way that I'll have evidence for the genuine niceness (Recorded Tutorial)

What I mean here and what I learned from the tutorial is that nurses might have been on their best behaviour when I observed them and this was what they aspired to most of the time. But this might not have been the way they behaved when I was not present. Their request for me not to record these forbidden data was perhaps their wish to hide the ugliness (Goffman, 1976a, 1976b). Yet this episode also suggested that they trusted me to know that they were showing bad behaviour. These acts of editing out and editing in allowed me to push the idea that niceness might be recognized as surface niceness or staged niceness, which the ethnomethodological gaze could not make visible.

Analytic Moments

Reflexivity also played a role in helping me choose my methodology: acting as an aide to the *analytic moment.* I was well in the process of data analysis in year 3. I was strongly influenced by Sacks' paper 'Doing being ordinary' (Sacks, 1992a). Sacks invites us to think of a person not as an 'ordinary person' but as someone who went about doing the things that most people did every day, for example, going to work, reading, eating or sleeping. For Sacks, being an 'ordinary' person was 'a job' (Sacks, 1992b, p. 217). 'Ordinariness' was to be found in the most mundane, seen but unnoticed and the tiniest activities. I was particularly interested in how the apparently unimportant and the most ordinary features of talk which we took for granted in our everyday life could be studied in a methodical way so that mundane talk such as 'hello', 'how do you do?' might be understood as the outcome of a rational, orderly procedure for the participants.

The diary's next entry raised the important implication for my choice of methodology and my concern to capture the seen but unnoticed features of what I observed in the field.

> Attended an ethnography study day at the RCN. Professor (...) opened the meeting by advising us to 'develop lateral thinking' (don't we know that?). 'Need to focus on details of features of everyday life' (we know that too, thank you very much!). 'Needed to be like Sherlock Homes, not

> Dr. Watson who could never see any clues' (this is interesting), 'need to look for unnoticed clues' (now let me think, who says this first? Garfinkel?). I asked him what analytic tool one could use to analysis all these details, he said he had none! 'Well, what can I say….?' (Research Diary Li, 2002a)

After reading through several key books on methodology that were potentially appropriate for my research topic, I narrowed down the available choices and decided to go for a combined ethnomethodological ethnographic approach (Li, 2002a, 2002b). This approach is both interpretive and inductive. Ethnography (like the work of Dr. Watson) provides clues for ethnomethodologists (like Sherlock Holmes) to investigate our social world. I felt that this approach was appropriate for my research topic. I was not just interested in how my participants explained or saw things like psychosocial care exclusively, but I was also using conversation analysis (CA) to demonstrate how nurses do psychosocial care in talk and interaction. This analytic approach enabled me to act like Sherlock Holmes but assisted by an 'internal' Dr. Watson to look for immediate evidence for locally produced, naturally accountable phenomena in palliative settings. It enabled me to make visible all the seen but unnoticed features in the daily interaction between palliative care nurses and patients (Li, 2002a, 2002b). It allowed the data to 'speak' to me rather than allowing theoretical concepts to influence my category generation. Through the application of the 'ethnomethodological gaze', I discovered my key construct and thesis concerning symbiotic niceness (Li, 2004).

Reflexivity also assisted me to deal with the messy reality of the literature review as this diary extract shows:

> Reading, reading and more reading! My data suggests that I ought to read Wittgenstein and Schutz! Is this really necessary? The trouble is if you don't read the literature, you can't discuss your findings in the context of other empirical studies. (Research Diary Li, 2002a)

When I made this diary entry above, I had already spent a whole year reading around the topic of psychosocial care in the palliative care context. I had also started to analyse my first batch of data. I was going into the areas of medicalization, total pain (Saunders & Baines, 1983) and the sociology of emotions and the body. At the time, I realized that I was going too wide and that I would have to cut out a big bulk of my literature review. This took some courage! The upgrade examiners (Upgrade Report 15 December 1999) helped me to do this. My research question 'What does it mean to do psychosocial care?' (Li, 2002a, 2002b) was far too broad to be a doctoral thesis and I had to refine my research question. I returned to my data and went through it like Sherlock Holmes looking for minute and unnoticed clues. I needed to establish a link between theory and data (Nadin & Cassell, 2006; Silverman, 2010b). However, I was still at a loss as to what my theoretical and analytical focuses were. More worryingly, my interest in psychosocial care was not directly related to the data analysis, which focused on the co-performance of niceness (Li, 2002a, 2002b).

Then at one particular tutorial, something suddenly clicked and my thesis was born. Silverman (2010b) said that a research topic (problem) 'rarely came out of the blue' (p. 31) but that it was given to us by supervision. This was an exchange between (SL) and my supervisor (C):

> C: being nice .....is a huge feature of these nurses' work, all right
> S: er
> C: they're terribly nice to you
> S: ah yes
> C: I am terribly struck by that ...yeah they do it very well (S: yeah) they do it effectively at being nice and the patients seem to say how nice they were
> S: that's right
> C: they've effectively got the patients saying everyone is so nice, they do it for you, relatives and patients, they do it to each other you know you could turn your thesis into that, that seems to me a lot of social psychosocial care actually is basically about being nice (Taped Tutorial two).

So I became interested in how people did the business of being nice, how they (nurses and doctors) did that through their talk. I began to find that psychosocial care was about being nice, and that it was enacted in emotional labour through the doing of niceness. The seed of my thesis was evidently planted in this tutorial (Li, 2002a, 2002b). Early in my

PhD journey, I had been diverted from where I should be going; I had lost my way and had to change direction. Reflexivity in this instance involved questioning and thinking about my theoretical choices, through actions of reading and re-reading, narrowing down, backtracking, discarding and refocusing I discovered my central thesis (Li, 2002a, 2002b).

My Personal Journey

The PhD journey was an emotional journey of personal learning where I used a reflexive attitude to manage emotions. I illustrate these emotional moments through describing three points where emotions were overwhelming. The first point I have called the 'lowest point':

> 'We discussed SL's literature review, on which a great deal of work has been done. I gave SL written comments on this and told her of my concerns that at present this would not reach the standard required for an MPhil or PhD. (Annual Progress Report)

The bottom of my PhD world fell out when I received the above report from my supervisor. This report concerned my first piece of work—the dreaded literature review. I edited out the following diary entry from my published dairies (Li, 2001, 2002a, 2002b, 2003; Li & Seale, 2007a) because, like the palliative care nurses who did not want me to report ugly moments, I too wanted to hide an ugly moment (Goffman, 1976a, 1976b). This was what I wrote on the day I received this report:

> 'I felt so utterly ashamed and worthless. How dared I, doing a PhD? I am not up to scratch! I can't even write! Damn me, damn you and damn the lot!' (Unpublished Research Diary).

Looking back, I was angry. My pride was damaged. My beloved father died in May 1997. I was at the lowest point of my research journey. I felt extremely angry; I hated myself and I hated him (my supervisor) (Li & Seale, 2007a). I hated everything. I ripped up this report furiously and went into hiding. I did not want to have any contact with anyone, including my supervisor. I withdrew into my own little world of self-centredness and apathy. There were many sympathetic emails from my supervisor who asked how I was getting on and making suggestions. I called this 'supportive questioning'. It was then that I decided to pick up the fragments of the ripped report (which I fortunately retained). I read the comments again and realized that they were not bad at all and that I could work on them. I asked myself: 'Why had I reacted in that foolish and childish way?' My wounds were healing and I bounced back with renewed energy and enthusiasm. I learned to take everything in my stride. I decided that I would chew over my supervisor's comments and learn from them. If I slipped back down, I would climb back up again immediately, as my diary entry showed below:

> 'Just as I thought. I nearly reached the top of the mountain only to slip right back down and a long way down to the bottom! Comments from Clive constructive. Must climb back up fast! A journey I must take!' (Research Diary Li, 2002a)

The outcome of my decision to carry on in spite of this adversity was that I realized that I could improve and produce a competent piece of literature review. I decided to resurface. I earned the following comments from my supervisor at a tutorial session (C my supervisor, S is SL):

> 'C: my overall feeling with all this is that this is really very much on the right track now, you know nicely expressed, you are looking at something interesting
> S: yeah I love it too I am glad
> C: good! I mean I am really pleased with your writing cos I know it's been really a struggle for you
> C: it does seem now you are on course now' (Recorded Tutorial 2)

The second emotional point occurred after my successful PhD viva. I was now a Doctor of Philosophy; thus my mission was accomplished, as my diary entry below showed:

> Examiner: 'Congratulations, Sarah. Dr. Li, you can now celebrate and sleep well tonight. Once again, congratulations and well done!' (Research Diary Li, 2003)

The final point was a *post script* as I reflected on the meaning my PhD had for me in the context of my personal history:

> I had a mission and this mission became all the more wanting as my darling father lay dying. For him I did this and for him I succeeded. Rest in peace now, Dad. (Research Diary Li, 2004)

Reflexivity for me involved reflecting, supportive questioning through emotional actions of ripping up, feeling fury and anger then picking up, hiding and withdrawing, resurfacing and bouncing back, slipping back and climbing up, looking back and moving on. Through these reflections and actions, I overcame this emotional impasse.

Strategies for Reflexivity in Field Research

I have shown the strategies I took to act on reflexivity at four critical moments of reflexivity. These strategies for practicing reflexivity enabled me to resolve and dissolve interactional troubles in the field and included:

- Reducing interactional distance by writing about resistances and troubles during fieldwork
- Censoring-self, which meant watching myself and watching others' reactions to me
- Fine-tuning the messy reality of theoretical and methodological questions to make my thesis doable and being brave to change direction
- Seeking active support from social networks and friends

Conclusion

In this chapter, I have contextualized and made visible the ambiguous concepts of 'self-dissolution', 'self-criticism' and 'self-application' (Beck et al., 1994) introduced in the beginning of this chapter. An examination of my doctoral research diary illustrates what reflexivity actually looks like. In line with other writers (Finlay, 2002; Nadin & Cassell, 2006;

Engward & Davis, 2015; Malaurent & Avison, 2017), reflexivity in this study involved deliberate acts of feeling, self-questioning, thinking, reflecting and emotional experience. The ethnomethodological gaze enabled a particular way of seeing. It helped me to identify additional acts of reflexivity: remembering and acting on that thinking (Nadin & Cassell, 2006). I do not intend what I have said to be treated as representative or applicable across all research contexts, as what I have written about is personal and subjective. My intention has been to provide a picture of what reflexivity looked like in practice during my journey to a PhD.

References

Alvesson, M., & Skoldberg, K. (2009). *Reflexive methodology. New vistas for qualitative research*. London: Sage.

Arber, A. (2006). Reflexivity: A Challenge for the researcher as practitioner? *Journal of Research in Nursing, 11*(2), 147–157.

Beck, U., Giddens, A., et al. (1994). Replies and critiques. In U. Beck, A. Giddens, & S. Lash (Eds.), *Reflexive modernization. Politics, traditions and aesthetics in the modern social order* (Chap. 4, pp. 174–215). London: Polity Press.

Borg, S. (2001). The research journal: A tool for promoting and understanding researcher development. *Learning Teaching Research, 5*(2), 156.

Buscatto, M. (2016). Practising reflexivity in ethnography. In D. Silverman (Ed.), *Qualitative research* (Chap. 9, pp. 137–151). London: Sage.

Coffey, A. (1999). *The ethnographic self*. London: Sage.

Engin, M. (2011). Research diary: A tool for scaffolding. *International Journal of Qualitative Methods, 10*(3), 296–306.

Engward, H., & Davis, G. (2015). Being reflexive in qualitative grounded theory: Discussion and application of a model of reflexivity. *Journal of Advance Nursing, 71*, 1530–1538.

Enosh, G. (2016). Reflexivity: The creation of liminal spaces-researchers, participants, and research encounters. *Qualitative Health Research, 26*(4), 578–584.

Finlay, L. (2002). Negotiating the swamp: The opportunity and challenge of reflexivity in research practice. *Qualitative Research, 2*(2), 209–230.

Foucault, M. (1963). *The birth of the clinic. An archaeology of medical perception*. London: Tavistock.

Garfinkel, H. (1967). *Studies in ethnomethodology*. Englewood Cliffs: Prentice Hall.

Garfinkel, H. (1992). Doing 'being ordinary'. In H. Sacks (Ed.), *Lectures on conversation* (Vol. 2). Oxford: Blackwell.

Goffman, E. (1967). *Interaction ritual. Essay on face-to-face behaviour*. London, Fakenham, and Reading: Penguin Books.

Goffman, E. (1976a). The nature of deference and demeanour. *American Anthropologist, 58*, 473–502.

Goffman, E. (1976b). *The presentation of self in everyday life*. Harmondsworth: Penguin Books.

Hammersley, M., & Atkinson, P. (1983). *Ethnography. Principles in practice*. London and New York: Routledge.

Hertz, R. (1997). *Reflexivity and voice*. Thousand Oaks, CA: Sage.

Kirk, J., & Miller, M. L. (1986). *Reliability and validity in qualitative research*. Newbury Park, London, and New Delhi: Sage.

Li, S. (1985). *Analysis of nursing environment using critical incidences of dying*. Unpublished B.Ed Research Project, University of Sussex, Sussex.

Li, S. (2001). My research diary: First year. *Current Research Newsletter*. Department of Sociology, Goldsmith's College, University of London, November (16): 15–18.

Li, S. (2002a). My research diary (Continued). *Current Research Newsletter*. Department of Sociology, Goldsmith's College, University of London, June (17): 8–10.

Li, S. (2002b). *Symbiotic niceness: A study of psychosocial care in palliative care settings*. PhD thesis. Goldsmith's College, University of London, London: 300.

Li, S. (2003). My research diary (The Grand Finale!). *Current Research Newsletter*. Department of Sociology, Goldsmith's College, University of London, March (18): 8–11.

Li, S. (2004). 'Symbiotic niceness': Constructing a therapeutic relationship in psychosocial palliative care. *Social Sciences & Medicine, 58*(12), 2571–2583.

Li, S. (2005). Doing criticism in symbiotic niceness: A study of palliative care nurses' talk. *Social Sciences & Medicine, 60*(9), 1949–1959.

Li, S. & C. Seale (2007a). Just you, me and the PhD. *The Times Higher Education Supplement*, p. 21. London.

Li, S., & Seale, C. (2007b). Learning to do qualitative data analysis: An observational study of PhD work. *Qualitative Health Research, 17*(10), 1442–1452.

Li, S., & Seale, C. (2007c). Managing criticism in PhD Supervision. *Studies in Higher Education, 32*(4), 511–526.

Li, S., & Seale, C. (2008). Acquiring a sociological identity: An observational study of a PhD project. *Sociology, 42*(5), 971–986.
Malaurent, J. & D. Avison (2017). Reflexivity: A third essential 'R' to enhance interpretive field studies. *Information & Management* (Available online 20 February 2017).
May, T., & Perry, B. (2010). *Social research and reflexivity. Content, consequences and context*. London: Sage.
Nadin, S., & Cassell, C. (2006). The use of a research diary as a tool for reflexive practice. *Qualitative Research in Accounting & Management, 3*(2), 208–217.
Potter, S. (2006). Academic writing. In S. Potter (Ed.), *Doing postgraduate research* (Chap. 6, pp. 114–150). London: Sage.
Rapley, T. (2007). *Doing conversation, discourse and document analysis*. Los Angeles: Sage.
Sacks, H. (1992a). Doing 'being ordinary'. In J. M. Atkinson & J. Heritage (Eds.), *Structure of social action: Studies in conversation analysis* (pp. 513–529). Cambridge: Cambridge University Press.
Sacks, H. (1992b). *Lectures on conversation* (Vol. 2). Oxford: Blackwell.
Saunders, C., & Baines, M. (1983). *Living with dying, the management of terminal illness*. Oxford: Oxford University Press.
Silverman, D. (2010a). Evaluating qualitative research. In D. Silverman (Ed.), *Doing qualitative research* (Chap. 16, pp. 202–308). London: Sage.
Silverman, D. (2010b). Quality in qualitative research. In D. Silverman (Ed.), *Doing qualitative research* (Chap. 15, 3rd ed., pp. 268–289). London: Sage.
Silverman, D. (2010c). The research experience 1. In D. Silverman (Ed.), *Doing qualitative research* (Chap. 3, 3rd ed., pp. 17–42). London: Sage.
Singnal, N. & R. Jeffrey (2008). Qualitative research skill workshop. A facilitator's reference manual. London. 2017. Retrieved from http://oer.educ.cam.ac.uk
Sudnow, D. (1967). *Passing on*. London and New York: Prentice Hall.

Sarah Li is an honorary research fellow at Kingston University and St George's, University of London, Faculty of Health, Social Care & Wellbeing, UK. Sarah has conducted research in palliative care, mental health and care of older people. She was awarded her Ph.D. in 2002 from Goldsmiths, University of London.

3

Emotions in the Field: Research in the Infertility Clinic

Helen T. Allan

Introduction

In this chapter, I draw on the findings of an ethnographic study of a British fertility unit to explore the role of emotions in fertility nursing practice. The study was undertaken because I was interested in why fertility nursing had been ignored in the literature on assisted reproductive technologies. I was interested in the contribution of nurses to the field of assisted reproduction and to the delivery of nursing care in an infertility unit. The study focused on the experiences of infertility for patients and nurses, and the implications of these experiences for the day-to-day management of care. My findings suggested that the expression of caring behaviours by nurses depended on their use of space within the clinic and that nurses, working mostly in the public spaces of the clinic, used these spaces to distance themselves from patients' emotions. The organisation of the clinic into public and private spaces enabled the management of potentially disruptive emotions of both nurses and the patients they cared for (Allan, 2001, 2002).

H.T. Allan (✉)
Department of Adult, Child, Midwifery, Middlesex University, London, UK

H.T. Allan, A. Arber (eds.), *Emotions and reflexivity in Health and Social Care Field Research*, https://doi.org/10.1007/978-3-319-65503-1_3

Background to the Study

Infertility is a major concern internationally, with an estimated incidence of 9% worldwide (ESHRE, 2014) although figures for the UK estimate it might be as high as 15% (HFEA, 2013). Fertility treatments such as in vitro fertilisation (IVF) and intra-cytoplasmic sperm injection (ICSI) allow many people to achieve parenthood with over 60,000 cycles of IVF being performed annually in the UK alone (HFEA, 2015). Success rates vary considerably due to age and diagnosis, but overall 17,041 cycles result in live births p.a., that is a 25.6% success rate using a woman's fresh eggs (HFEA, 2015). Assisted reproductive technologies (ARTs) account for 2% of all live births p.a., and the majority of IVF/ICSI cycles involve couples using their own eggs and sperm (HFEA, 2015).

At the same time as the technological potential to investigate and diagnose infertility has increased, success rates have remained relatively low (Bennet & Templeton, 1995). There is much that remains a puzzle in relation to infertility and its biomedical management. In addition, the availability of infertility treatments has been described as unfair; infertility treatments are not funded fully and access to any treatments has been described as a 'postcode lottery' (Souter, 1997; www.rcog.org.uk, 2004). Interventions such as donor gametes, surrogacy and sex selection problematise the meaning of conception and the social and legal status of the embryo; they raise questions about whether an embryo is human and 'who' society accepts as human, and therefore whether that person is entitled to fundamental human rights and protection from harm.

Fertility nurses provide outpatient services to couples and single women seeking either a diagnosis of their fertility problem or help with ARTs. Fertility nurses are employed in NHS and private clinics and consider themselves a sub-speciality of gynaecology or women's health nursing (Allan, 2009a, 2009b; Allan & Mounce, 2016.

The Role of Emotions in Research

Fineman (2004) argues that descriptions of organisations are often bland and do not paint a picture of the emotional component of working life. This is surprising given that the British National Health Service has been called the 'keep death at bay service' (Obholzer & Zagier Roberts, 1994, p. 171). This feature of health professionals' work, the keeping death at bay, engenders emotions which are also kept at bay, or unconsciously defended against as painful to bring to conscious awareness except at certain times, such as the actual death of a patient (Armstrong & Rustin, 2014; Huffington, Halton, Armstrong, & Pooley, 2004). Although overtly expressed emotions can be problematic in British hospitals as they can disrupt the sentimental order of the clinic (Irwin, 2002; Wells, 2000). In fact, Menzies (1970) rather famously argued that the highly structured hierarchy characteristic of British nursing had emerged as an unconscious means to defend against the anxiety in everyday nursing relationships with patients (Allan, 2009a, 2009b).

Fineman suggests that the study of emotions at work allows two processes to emerge. Firstly, people, their behaviours and the effects of those behaviours come to the fore and become the focus of study. Secondly, emotions are understood to be the main medium through which people act and interact. My findings showed that the organisation of nursing work was anything but bland; the organisation of nursing work and the unit was shaped by the anxiety raised by the emotions evoked by the experience of being infertile and caring for infertile people (Allan, 2001, 2002, 2009a, 2009b). Comparing sources of data using observations and interviews revealed that there were discrepancies between the narratives nurses and patients told about caring and nursing work and the reality of practice. For example, in their narratives, patients identified caring with nurses rather than doctors or receptionists, and believed that nurses understood the patient's experience. The nurse's role was to work with the doctor, to care and be there to support patients. Participants (patients and nurses) saw nurses as closer to patients in the sense that nurses understood what patients were experiencing and could communicate with them because of their personal qualities, the types of activities they carried out for patients as they arrived and the intimacy of their relationships.

However, in observing their relationships with nurses in the clinic, I found that these data contradicted what I observed nurses doing. The nurses did not generally accompany women into the doctor's room and did not know what happened in consultations because they were not present during the consultations. The women had few opportunities to be intimate as they had no contact other than social contact with the nurses. Comparison of data during fieldwork enabled multiple stories and realities to emerge, and for the blandness of organisational life to be peeled away and the complexities of practice revealed. However, these data were difficult emotionally to witness and process as I shall discuss later in this chapter.

The Research Process

I used an ethnographic approach informed by feminist research (e.g. built upon a belief that research could be empowering and woman-focused). The choice of this methodology emerged from my epistemological starting point that research should be a reflexive process informed by my position as an infertile woman as well as an investigation of the aims of the study (Coffey, 1999; Hall & Stevens, 1991; Webb, 1993). My starting point was informed by research debates around the use of reflexivity and giving voice to individual's experience in the field (Brooks, 1997; Finlay, 2002; Frost, 2016; McCarl Neilson, 1990; Stanley & Wise, 1993; Walter, 1998; Watts, 2008; Weller & Caballero, 2009). Given that I wanted to uncover staff and patients' views and experiences of fertility nursing, ethnography offered a way to observe social processes and culture such as medical consultations and procedures (Porter, 1998). The research relationships developed during fieldwork offered the potential for change in nursing practice through reflection with staff in the field (Skeggs, 1994). The nurses were observed to mainly provide chaperoning,[1] ensuring the clinic ran on time, helped doctors perform medical investigations, tested urine and weighed patients. Two research nurses performed a more advanced role, undertaking donor insemination and post-coital examinations and tests.

Participant observation data comprised my field notes taken during and after observations in the field. I would write notes during short breaks outside the unit and then, when I had left the field, or shortly after, record them in more detail; I would transcribe all the notes taken that week fully at the weekend. These notes recorded actions or work carried out in the unit while I was present as well as reflections I had about the observations of, and informal conversations I had with staff and patients. It included what I called 'noises off', where I was not present but could either overhear or was told about an incident at a later stage. The participant observation and field notes formed a larger proportion of the data collected than I had expected as staff used the opportunity to talk to me informally during periods of observation. These data allowed a variety of observations on the clinic work, the experience of infertility and the emotions engendered in myself and others. Gradually, as I became more confident and better at recalling events during participant observation, I realised that I had been trying to stop myself 'going native' or becoming immersed in the social world of the clinic (Hammersley & Atkinson, 1983). However, I realised that I was already a 'native', rather than being at risk of going native (Ganesh, 1993; Kleinman & Copp, 1993); that is, I was both a researcher and a participant, with my own experiences of being a nurse, a researcher and an infertile woman.

The Experience of Positioning Myself in the Research

Initially, I found the role of privileged observer (Wolcott, 1988) helpful in suggesting the position of participant observer. I was privileged because of the staff's knowledge that I was a nurse tutor and had past relationships with some of the nurses (Hammersley & Atkinson, 1983; Skeggs, 1994; Stacey, 1988). My position as a nurse tutor could have influenced nurses' interactions with me. I had taught many of them in my role as a link tutor before starting data collection. While this facilitated entry, at times they might have deferred to me in a clinical situation, which I wanted to avoid. However, these insights did not fully describe the complexities of participant observation in familiar settings, and I found Peberdy's paper on participant observation more useful (1993) in capturing the realities of choices presented to the ethnographer in participant observation. She argues that because human observation involves people, the question about involvement in relation to observation/participation becomes 'not so much, should I become involved?' but rather 'what level and style of involvement and participation is appropriate, useful and acceptable in this particular situation?' (1993, p. 48).

I also like Savage's discussion of participative observation here, drawing on ideas of embodiment to suggest that we are reflexively the observation we observe (1995). The style of involvement and participation was as an additional person assisting at a procedure, rather than performing as a member of the team. It was also influenced by ethical considerations. If things were busy or the need arose, I would occasionally do a pregnancy test, hold someone's hand or clear away a trolley, but I preferred to assist a nurse rather than 'be' a nurse (active participant). This degree of involvement provided experience of doing the nursing which I could then reflect on (Jackson, 1989; Savage, 1995). However, I became aware that I was not answering the question honestly: 'what level and style of involvement and participation is appropriate, useful and acceptable in this particular situation?'. I began to record feelings arising from being a participant observer in my diary and reflexivity became an established, meaningful part of my study when I realised that the study raised emotions for me which needed to be managed.

I think my reluctance to be more involved and the accompanying need to stand back stemmed from my own infertility. My infertility aroused feelings that made me identify with the patients undergoing procedures and I preferred to be, at least partly distant (this was particularly acute when I was going through a period of IVF myself). However, I kept most of these feelings and thoughts out of my academic supervision. Yet, as Walkerdine, Lucey, and Meldoy (2001) suggest, this avoidance had an impact which I have described to friends as 'putting my head above the parapet' when presenting my work. I did not do as Walkerdine et al. (2001) suggest: use those personal feelings openly. Instead I used professional feelings from my positioning as a nurse and researcher collecting data in the field. Also undertaking the study was making me feel troubled by the experiences I was seeing and hearing. After the patient interviews, I was often sad and hopeless, and I used the diary to separate my own feelings and those expressed by patients during interview. I was identifying with the women and their experience as in practice I had been through what they were going through although I felt unable to share this with them at the time.

Baszanger and Dodier (1997) call the decision about which role to adopt as participant observer as finding the right distance between the observer and participant. These concerns and feelings could have produced an ethnography that used my experiences as a patient as a resource for analysis along with the experiences of my participants (Callaway, 1992; Stanley & Wise, 1993; Walkerdine et al. 2001). However, in this study I was predominantly positioning myself as a researcher who used past experiences to shape the research and to make an interpretative reading of the data (Rudge, 1996). I realised during the period of participant observation that I was reflexively using my own emotions in the field to be responsive to the emotions of others and I then used these insights to analyse the data, as Kleinman and Copp suggest (1993). During fieldwork, I began to observe how the experiences of infertility and the beliefs shaping these experiences affected the expression and management of emotions by staff and patients in the unit.

Murray Parkes (1998) has argued that members of the healthcare professions are affected by grief during their work with different types of loss and chronic sorrow, but that they rarely acknowledge their feelings and the effects these can have on their practice or themselves. Little attempt is made to apply these concepts of loss and grief in fertility nursing or to understand the impact emotions and loss have on fertility work. It seemed that the staff and patients managed infertility in ways to avoid acknowledging the loss and pain that are part of the experience as well as its medical management.

At this point, I started to record two sets of notes: one written from participant observation as field notes, and another a diary. The diary helped me to achieve a degree of reflexivity in representing the different voices in the data, i.e. including my voice as a participant and a researcher. Indeed, Kleinman and Copp (1993) argue that it is the degree of reflexivity and openness to emotions in fieldwork that produce rich ethnographic data by using the emotions elicited and observed during fieldwork.

However, this decision to have field notes and to keep a diary to aid reflexivity now looks more complicated than it seemed at the time. Walkerdine et al.'s (2001) account of using psychoanalytic approaches to reflexivity in fieldwork would see this decision to 'split' my personal feelings off from my 'research' data as a positivist spin revealing a desire to split off my feelings from my field notes. They would suggest (imagining a conversation with them in my supervision) that I should have used my feelings explicitly in the research as data. Instead I hid my feelings from my supervisors and was anxious to keep them out of the analysis. Only when feelings were insights into the data, did I utilise them. For example, I acknowledged and used feelings of social isolation while observing in the waiting room where patients waited for up to an hour for their appointments to inform my analysis of the use of space in the clinic as defences against the anxiety of infertility. But I did not acknowledge my feelings of sadness at my own infertility when I felt sad listening to interview recordings but kept myself firmly focused on the interviewees' words and feelings.

I observed clinical interactions between patients and medical staff in the consulting rooms during discussion of treatments or results, or procedures such as post-coital vaginal examinations and intrauterine inseminations with either donor or husband's sperm. Observation of these procedures raised potential ethical issues for me as an observer and as a nurse in a dual role. I was granted ethical clearance to observe on the basis that I was there as a participant observer—that is, to assist if necessary on the basis of my research role, not as a nurse. Therefore, I had to gain verbal consent during each period of observation to remind patients, and staff that I was there as a researcher, not as a nurse. I also observed interactions between patients and nurses that took place in the Sister's office in the assisted conception unit (ACU) and the consulting room in the research clinic. Social interactions were observed in the corridor, waiting room and the reception areas of the clinic. The social interactions were mainly between nurses and patients in the waiting room and corridor, as doctors and counsellors were rarely seen outside of their private consulting rooms during clinic. The main point here is that patients saw doctors in private, and nurses saw patients in the more public areas of the clinic. It occurred to me then that perhaps nurses were not seen as important enough to be allocated any private space.

Using a feminist psychoanalytic approach, I argued that the experience of infertility is so powerful emotionally that caring and non-caring were strategies used by staff to manage emotions, which threatened the social order of the clinic (Allan, 2000). Traditional relationships between nursing and medicine which are shaped by gendered caring resulted in nurses 'nursing the clinic and doctor' rather than nursing the patient as this extract from my field notes shows:

> Lizzie showed patients in and responded to the bell when Dr Thomas rang for attention. She also brought him in a cup of tea at 3pm and hassled him about running late—knocked on the door and reminded him that there was a queue of patients to see.

These findings have been reported in more detail elsewhere (Allan, 2001, 2002).

Data from both participant observation and interviews suggested that nurses were emotionally distant from patients. Patients did not know the names of the nurses looking after them or, indeed, spend any longer than five minutes interacting with nurses during the course of a clinic. Patients did not acknowledge the contradictory nature of their descriptions of the nurse–patient relationship (emotionally close) and the reality of their experiences (emotionally distant). As I continued participant observation and interviewing, my understanding of nursing changed as two discrepancies emerged from the different sources of data. I should say that, at the time, my observation of these discrepancies was emotional; that is, I felt the discrepancies in my body before I understood them. However, during supervision after re-reading my diary, my analysis of the data was more from a rational, logical stance, what Walkerdine et al. (2001) describe as the positivist approach to reflexivity, which retains an understanding of reflexivity as a cognitive process rather than an emotional one.

The 'Discrepancies'

In my data, I found discrepancies between what patients said they expected from a 'good nurse' and how they talked about their relationships with nurses. The following extract was pretty common across the interview data:

> HA: Right. What sort of relationship have you built up with the nurses?
> PT: Oh I've got to know them a lot now and they've got to know me. If I phone and I've got a query they know me now. So that's quite good 'cos I can go straight to them now and not have to go through the receptionist. They can help me more than the receptionist can.
> HA: And do you know them?
> PT: I know Mirabelle better than Gloria 'cos when I first came here she was the only nurse I saw and I built up a relationship with her.
> HA: And can you think of a particular occasion when she's helped you?
> PT: Oh Gawd!
> Turns to her husband.
> PT: She's took my blood pressure hasn't she? Um....she gets all me bits and pieces together. She's always been all right towards me. The other one I don't know she's ever done anything for me.

What I saw here was the way in which the patient says she is known by and knows the nurse Mirabelle but even so struggles to explain what care she has received from her. However, Mirabelle is accessible, and she takes observations and they seem to have a relationship as they are known to each other. What I infer from this exchange and others like it in my data is the discrepancy between what is expected or idealised in a nurse and the reality of the contact or relationship.

Another discrepancy arose between what staff described as caring in interviews and their expressed views of infertility and infertile patients. I arrived at this understanding in the analysis through a comparison of the data in my field notes and transcripts and coding of interviews. Writing in my diary about my feelings was a way of legitimising my feelings by turning them into thoughts. It was a turning point in my analysis as it allowed me to critique existing literature on the role of emotions in practice and to develop a feminist psychoanalytic understanding of gendered relations in the context of nurses caring for infertile women. This insight enabled me to understand how both myself as a researcher and the nurses in the clinic were defending ourselves against anxiety aroused by the expression of strong emotion in the clinic.

As I interviewed staff and read transcripts of interviews while continuing to take field notes, I had to try hard not to judge the nurses in a professional way as a nurse, but to explore how the context in which nursing took place shaped the caring that emerged. For me, at this time, it was a turning point as I realised that I had expectations of the nurses that were not being met and I began to question myself in relation to the nurses observed behaviour, which seemed non-caring. The following field note data expresses a level of discomfort with how staff treated patients in a way that lacked etiquette and kindness:

> When you sit in the corridor opposite the lift on the second floor, everyone coming to that part of the hospital looks at you. It is not as private as the ACU even though Shirley said its better because it doesn't feel like an outpatient department. Shirley's door is closed and locked and has a notice saying 'Don't ring the bell…Sister will attend to you when its your turn. Please fill in the pink form before Sister calls you'. You wait staring at the lift doors. This feels quite isolating because there's no receptionist to say hello to although Shirley comes out occasionally and says hello on her way to the sperm bank. Dr Winter opened the door today and said aggressively 'who's next?' She looked at me and I said 'I'm not a patient'. Patient said 'I am'. Then she barked 'have you filled in your pink form?' No. 'Well, fill it in then' and closed the door. The patient did so and a few minutes later Dr Winter opened the door and said 'Done? Come in then'.

I was (and still am) struck by several feelings in these data such as feeling isolated, feeling exposed, experiencing aggression from one of the doctors who barked at patients and feeling shut out by the closed doors. My diary writing helped me to reflect on my observations and interactions in my field notes and became a more personal record of my feelings. I remember quite clearly feeling very alone and, at the time, felt this was because as a researcher I was alone. But now, I can see that feeling alone also described my experiences of being 'alone' as an infertile woman in a fertile world. In my field notes I recorded my feelings, 'I saw this', 'I felt that', which helped me to separate my feelings and observations from those of the participants, to understand the relationship between the two as well as understand and interpret analytic notes. In addition to recording analytic notes I recorded my responses to the analytic notes in an attempt to keep feelings separate from thought. Below is an extract from my diary, which showed how separating the field notes from the diary helped me to analyse those emotions:

> When I observe situations where staff make judgments about infertile people I sometimes collude with staff and become an insider. In one case, a woman was described to me by Phoebe and Shula as 'pathological'. The overwhelming feeling in the consulting room after she had left was that the woman was being unreasonable. The staff could not empathise with her anxiety to have the treatment which was being cancelled due to the clinic shutting for Easter. She had been through the cycle, had been given the drugs but now the treatment cycle was being cancelled. At the time, I felt frustrated with her as they did. But writing up my diary and my notes for data analysis, repositioning myself as an outsider again, I saw why she was frustrated. She had lost two pregnancies and was prepared to go through 26 cycles of treatment to have a baby. But the staff were frustrated and exasperated and could not empathise. I wonder if the woman was labeled pathological to deal with these strong feelings? The strength of these negative feelings was evident when this woman conceived on her 26th treatment cycle. The news swept through the clinic like wild fire and staff were delighted that at last they did not have to 'face her in the clinic again'.

The relationship between participant observation data (recorded in field notes) analysis and interview data was the mechanism by which the turning point in my analysis emerged. While I understand Walkerdine et al.'s argument that I risked (2001) splitting off affect from thought, I felt at the time that I was able to feel the affect and reflect on that cognitively as part of analysis. The splitting of affect into field notes and a diary enabled my assisted thought, reflection and emotional expression. I would not deny that this process was at times a struggle. Walkerdine et al.

(2001) would suggest that the struggle with one's identity is inevitable. Using participant observation over a long period of time in order to immerse oneself in the field, combined with repeated informal and formal interviews, allowed me to analyse the data to understand the complexities of practice as well as to understand my own reactions to what I was seeing and hearing. Using the diary as part of reflexivity enabled insights into my own and other's emotions.

Reflexivity and Authority

Using reflexivity enabled me to see that the final ethnographic report is not necessarily the 'truth' as there are many realities. The final report or thesis is the researcher's representation; indeed, I have shaped and produced it in a knowing manner as someone with many identities as a feminist, a researcher, a clinician and an insider and outsider. My approach to authority is shaped by wider debates on this subject in both sociology (Atkinson, 1993; Enquix, 2014; Turner, 1991) and anthropology (Walter, 1995; Williams, 1990). Rudge (1996) argues that field notes reveal different voices, those of the researcher and the participants. Recording and analysing these voices reveals the researcher within the research and the effect of self on analysis. This is consistent with postmodern concerns with representing the different voices within research and the different identities produced in the field.

Strategies for Reflexivity in the Field

- Use your supervision for reflecting on emotions.
- Record your feelings every day in the field including the uncomfortable ones and discuss them in supervision.
- Be intuitive—don't rely on being able to articulate feelings but respond to bodily feelings and note them in your research diary.
- Be aware of one's sensitivities within the research setting and seek good support.

Conclusions

Understanding what reflexivity is and knowing how to be reflexive is not just a question of technique—although knowing how to and understanding what reflexivity is are important for the novice researcher to develop. Walkerdine et al. (2001) describe sharing the affects the emotions experienced. However, my feelings were at times difficult to discuss in supervision because the personal emotions were understood by myself to be inappropriate in the context of a PhD. This is a recurring theme in this book that emotions can be written out of the thesis and the study as something to be avoided in an academic context. However, Walkerdine et al.'s (2001) book *Growing Up Girl*, particularly Chap.4 'Working with Emotions', gives guidance on how to incorporate emotional literacy in academic work. I have tried to use this approach in my PhD supervisions as well as in other academic work (Allan, 2009a, 2009b; Allan, 2011). I think my reluctance to share my feelings from fieldwork with my supervisor says more about the research student's need to be in control in the face of much that is uncontrollable in fieldwork.

This chapter is based on a paper published in the *Journal of Nursing Research* in 2006 and is reproduced and updated for this book with permission from the publishers.

Notes

1. Chaperoning is a much underestimated nursing role, which encompasses *being with* as well as preserving patients' dignity in the face of the intimate gynaecological examination. I argue (Allan 2005) that it offers a containing of anxiety for women undergoing such examinations. It was valued by patients but not by managers seeking to find room to reduce staff costs. Allan H T (2005) Gender and embodiment in nursing: the role of the female chaperone in the infertility clinic *Nursing Inquiry* 12 (3) 175–183.

References

Allan, H. T. (2000). *Sister will see you now: Managing emotions in a fertility clinic.* Unpublished PhD thesis. Manchester University/Royal College of Nursing Institute.

Allan, H. T. (2001). Nursing the clinic and managing emotions in a fertility unit: Findings from an ethnographic study. *Nursing Inquiry, 8*, 51–60.

Allan, H. T. (2002). Nursing the clinic, being there, hovering: Ways of caring in a British fertility unit. *Journal of Advanced Nursing, 38*(1), 86–93.

Allan, H. T. (2009a). Emotions in check. *Nursing Standard, 23*(46), 61.

Allan, H. T. (2009b). *Managing intimacy and emotions in advanced fertility care: The future of nursing and midwifery roles.* London: M&K Publishing.

Allan, H. T. (2011). Using psycho-dynamic small group work in nurse education: Closing the theory-practice gap? *Nurse Education Today, 31*(5), 521–524.

Allan, H. T., & Mounce, G. (2016). The management of infertility in primary care. *Practice Nursing, 25*(1), 374–377.

Armstrong, D., & Rustin, M. (2014). *Social defenses against anxiety: Explorations in a paradigm* (Vol. 1). Tavistock Clinic Series. London: Karnac Books.

Atkinson, P. (1993). *Medical talk and medical work.* London: Routledge.

Baszanger, I., & Dodier, N. (1997). Ethnography: Relating the part to the whole. In D. Silverman (Ed.), *Qualitative research.* London: Sage.

Bennet, S., & Templeton, A. (1995). The epidemiology of infertility. In L. Meerabeau & J. Denton (Eds.), *Infertility nursing and caring* (pp. 42–55). London: Scutari Press.

Brooks, A. (1997). *Postfeminisms: Feminism, cultural theory and cultural forms.* London: Routledge.

Callaway, H. (1992). Ethnography and experience, gender implication in fieldwork and texts. In K. J. Okely & H. Callaway (Eds.), *Anthropology and autobiography* (pp. 30–49). London: Routledge.

Coffey, A. (1999). *The ethnographic self: Fieldwork and the representation of identity.* London: Sage.

Enquix, B. (2014). Negotiating the field: Rethinking ethnographic authority, experience and the frontiers of research. *Qualitative Research, 14*(1), 79–94.

European Society of Human Reproduction & Embryology (ESHRE). (2014). *ART fact sheet*, June 2014. Retrieved from http://www.eshre.eu/ESHRE/English/Guidelines-Legal/ART-fact-sheet/page.aspx/1061

Fineman, S. (2004). *Understanding emotion at work*. London: Sage.

Finlay, L. (2002). Negotiating the swamp: The opportunity and challenge of reflexivity in research practice. *Qualitative Research*. https://doi.org/10.1177/146879410200200205230

Frost, N. (2016). *Practising research: Why you're always part of the research even when you think you're not*. London: Palgrave.

Ganesh, K. (1993). Breaching the wall of difference: Fieldwork and a personal journey to Srivaikuntam, Tamilnadu. In D. Bell, P. Caplan, & W. J. Karim (Eds.), *Gendered fields: Women, men and ethnography* (pp. 128–142). London: Routledge.

Hall, J., & Stevens, P. (1991). Rigor in feminist research. *Advances in Nursing Sciences, 13*(3), 16–29.

Hammersley, M., & Atkinson, P. (1983). *Ethnography: Principles in practice*. London: Routledge.

Huffington, C., Halton, W., Armstrong, D., & Pooley, J. (2004). *Working below the surface: The emotional life of contemporary organisations*. Tavistock Clinic Series. London: Karnac Books.

Human Fertility & Embyrology Authority. (2013). *Latest UK IVF figures: 2013*. Retrieved January 5, 2015, from http://www.hfea.gov.uk/docs/HFEA_Fertility_Trends_and_Figures_2013.pdf

Human Fertility & Embryology Authority. (2015). Retrieved January 20, 2016, from www.Hfea.gov.org/AllabouttheHFEA

Irwin, R. (2002). *Psychosexual nursing*. London: Whurr Publishers, Ltd.

Jackson, M. (1989). *Paths towards a clearing*. Bloomington, IN: Indiana University Press.

Kleinman, S., & Copp, M. A. (1993). *Emotions and fieldwork*. Qualitative Research Methods Series, 28. London: Sage.

McCarl Neilson, J. (Ed.). (1990). *Feminist research methods*. Colorado: Westview Press.

Menzies, I. E. P. (1970). *The functioning of social systems as a defence against anxiety*. London: The Tavistock Institute of Human Relations.

Murray Parkes, C. (1998). Facing loss. *British Medical Journal, 316*, 1521–1524.

Obholzer, A., & Zagier Roberts, V. (1994). *The unconscious at work, individual and organisational stress in the human services*. London: Routledge.

Peberdy, A. (1993). Observing. In P. Shakespeare, D. Atkinson, & S. French (Eds.), *Reflecting on research practice* (pp. 47–57). Buckingham: Open University Press.

Porter, S. (1998). *Social theory and nursing practice*. London: Macmillan Press Ltd.

Rudge, T. (1996). (Re)writing ethnography: The unsettling questions for nursing research raised by post-structural approaches to the field. *Nursing Inquiry, 3*(3), 146–152.

Savage, J. (1995). *Nursing intimacy*. London: Scutari Press.

Skeggs, B. (1994). Situating the production of feminist ethnography. In M. Maynard & J. Purvis (Eds.), *Researching women's lives from a feminist perspective* (pp. 72–92). London: Taylor and Francis Ltd.

Souter, V. L. (1997). A survey of infertility practices in Scotland. *British Journal General Practice, 47*(424), 727–728.

Stacey, J. (1988). Can there be a feminist ethnography? *Women's Studies International Forum, 11*(1), 21–27.

Stanley, L., & Wise, S. (1993). *Breaking out again: Feminist ontology and epistemology* (New ed.). London: Routledge.

Turner, L. (1991). Feminism, femininity and ethnographic authority. *Women: A Cultural Review, 2*(3), 238–254.

Walkerdine, V., Lucey, H., & Meldoy, J. (2001). *Growing up girl. Psychosocial explorations of gender and class*. Basingstoke, UK: Palgrave.

Walter, L. (1995). Feminist anthropology? *Gender and Society, 9*(3), 272–288.

Walter, N. (1998). *The new feminism*. London: Virago Press.

Watts, J. H. (2008). Emotion, empathy and exit: Reflections on doing ethnographic qualitative research on sensitive topics. *Medical Sociology Online, 3*(2), 3–14.

Webb, C. (1993). Feminist research: Definitions, methodology, methods and evaluation. *Journal of Advanced Nursing, 18*(3), 416–423.

Weller, S., & Caballero, C. (2009). *Up close and personal: Relationship and emotions through and within research*. Working Paper No. 25, Family & Social Capital Research Group, South Bank University. ISBN 978-0-946786-59-6.

Wells, D. (2000). *Caring for sexuality in health and illness*. Edinburgh: Churchill Livingstone.

Williams, A. (1990). *Reflections on the making of an ethnographic text*. Studies in Sexual Politics No. 29. Manchester: Manchester University Press.

Wolcott, D. (1988). Ethnographic research in education. In R. M. Jaeger (Ed.), *Complementary methods for research in education*. Washington, DC: American Educational Research Association.

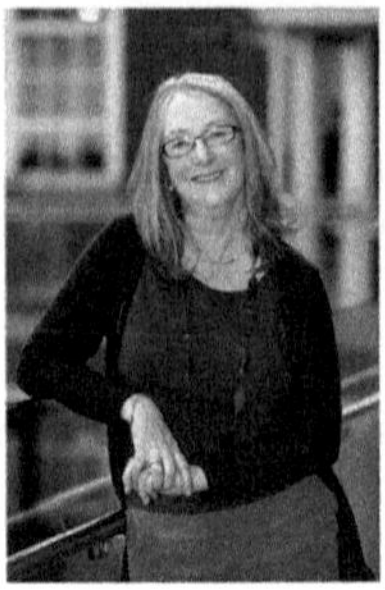

Helen T. Allan is Professor in Nursing at the Centre for Critical Research in Nursing & Midwifery, Middlesex University, London, UK. Helen was awarded her Ph.D. in 2000 from the Royal College of Nursing Institute/University of Manchester. Helen has supervised Ph.D. and clinical doctorates since 2002.

4

Managing the Dual Identity: Practitioner and Researcher

Anne Arber

Introduction

In this chapter, the focus is on what it means to have a dual identity as a practitioner and researcher. Moments when tension between the roles of researcher and practitioner were experienced are discussed. Some difficulties when managing the boundary between closeness and distance in terms of the observer and participant roles are highlighted as well as some challenges for the researcher with a dual identity. Keeping a marginal positioning on the boundary between the practitioner and researcher identities is not easy and enhancing credibility through methods of reflexive accounting is important when using qualitative methods. The lived experience of fieldwork will be explored, including insider and outsider identity management and how identity crises were managed and resolved. Reflexive practice is about recognising who we are and how we are part of the worlds we study.

A. Arber (✉)
University of Surrey, Guildford, UK

H.T. Allan, A. Arber (eds.), *Emotions and reflexivity in Health and Social Care Field Research*, https://doi.org/10.1007/978-3-319-65503-1_4

Reflexivity is characteristic of the ethnographic imagination and establishes the researchers' integrity, which is part of good ethnographic practice (Brewer, 1994). All ethnographic research involves ambiguities, missing materials and limitations within the field of study. It may be difficult to gain access to certain activities when gatekeepers control access or gatekeepers wish to monitor the research that is taking place and potentially influence the research in unexpected ways. Recently, this was experienced when conducting a focus group with patients and carers about their end-of-life care experiences. One of the nurses wished to be present in the focus group and it became apparent that the nurse wished to offer patients advice whereas the researcher wished to explore and understand patients' experience of symptoms. As this situation shows, there may be different interpretations of the meanings of what was asked, and why; of what was observed, spoken about or said. Researchers therefore have to be flexible but also careful and disciplined in their practice when documenting and writing up field experiences. Working reflexively enables the researcher to think about their actions and values during the research when producing data and analysing the data, and to view the beliefs they hold in the same way they view the beliefs of others (Gouldner, 1972; Seale, 1998).

In this chapter, I draw on ethnographic fieldwork from a study carried out within a UK hospice setting (Arber 2004). When designing the research, I was concerned with the sensitivity of the setting, where patients are generally extremely ill and dying. So the wish was to gather data with minimum disruption to work routines within the hospice. I was also concerned about avoiding the danger that my presence would interrupt the work of the staff and my presence as an observer would cause distress to staff and/or patients. I was interested in how hospice and palliative care staff talk about patients who have pain and how they worked with the concept of 'total pain'. The research design included audio recordings of palliative care team meetings and fieldwork concerned with observing staff during ward rounds and shadowing staff when visiting patients in their home. I sought to combine subjective and objective methods of data collection by combining participant observation with the audio recording of naturally occurring data collected in multidisciplinary team meetings.

Framing the Study: A Naturalistic Approach

I framed the study within the naturalistic paradigm of an ethnographic study. My intention was to spend time in the research field observing as much as I could of the action in relation to the problem of pain. The naturalistic approach to research includes attending to what informants tell you and beginning to understand what things mean to them (Gubrium & Holstein, 1997). One of the difficulties of the naturalistic approach is that it may be difficult to maintain any distance, as getting up close to the action and being involved in the action, one might overlook the more interesting aspects of what is going on (Gubrium & Holstein, 1997). Terms such as 'bracketing' and 'suspending' have been coined to alert the researcher to the issues of distance and the aim of objectivity when a researcher is studying one's own tribe for example (Pollner, 1987).

The issue of distance is important. As a nurse, I am familiar with the medical world, its specialised language and culture, and I felt at home in this world. This familiarity, I reasoned, might blind me to certain aspects of the setting that I took for granted. Thus, I felt I needed to get as close as I could to the action but to balance this by stepping back so that an eye is cast on how everyday realities are experienced (Gubrium & Holstein, 1997). It is suggested that to learn participants' meanings, we need to not only be reflexive about our own meanings but to attempt to 'flow' with the experiences in the world that is studied (Charmaz, 2004). Following Silverman (2001), data which are naturally occurring exist independently of the researcher's intervention; so to some extent these data have a degree of objectivity in that they are not researcher-provoked data. I felt that this combined approach to data collection would enable a balance between closeness and distance, incorporating a degree of subjectivity by participating and observing in the field (making field notes), balanced by collecting naturally occurring data that was audio recorded. This approach may shed light on the tacit and implicit that may not be easily shared as they are taken for granted (Charmaz, 2004).

Making Contact, Gaining Access and Acceptability

As an experienced practitioner in the field of cancer care, I had a network of existing contacts on which to draw to enable access to a hospice setting. However, I still felt concerned about whether I would gain access. Back (2002) describes a sense of trepidation when beginning research and worrying about contacting people. For example, Lawton (2000) an anthropologist, found initial access to a hospice setting difficult. However, once she gained the trust of the hospice professionals in the day care unit, she was granted free access within the hospice and successfully completed her research taking on the role of a volunteer. Hospice staff understandably feel protective toward their patients as they are usually very ill and dying.

As a researcher, there is a need to try out social positions in the field in order to facilitate access, establish rapport and gain trust as well as gaining information about the settings in which the research could take place with access to the unsaid, the taboo and unexpected (Miller & Glassner, 2004). My first point of contact was a local hospice. However, the hospice was going through major organisational change and my key contact (a senior nurse) had left the hospice suddenly. I made a decision not to pursue entry to this hospice as my key contact was unavailable. Within the second hospice, I approached the senior nurse who was interested in my research. She was prepared to act as my sponsor and I was given direct access to the hospice Medical Director. Gatekeepers have the power to grant or block access within a setting and they have expectations about the ethnographer's identity and intentions. In this setting, I felt that the gatekeepers were keen to sponsor my research. It is important to put out feelers and test out whether the host community sees the researcher as an expert and thus someone to be welcomed or as a critic and therefore unwelcome (Hammersley & Atkinson, 1995). At this stage, I believe I was being positioned toward the expert status rather than the critic as I had built up a good relationship with the senior nurse.

I was invited in to the hospice to meet with the Medical Director and he showed me around the hospice and introduced me to many of the staff. When we went into the community team office, I realised I knew one of the community nurses. She greeted me in a friendly manner and the Medical Director said, 'She speaks well of you. This is payback time'. I realised that this link may help my acceptability with other staff and smooth my entrance to doing the research. Lawton (2000) describes how once she had developed good rapport with day care staff, it was then easy to set up her second project within the hospice as the hospice staff had heard positive reports about her fieldwork.

I had two concerns about going into the palliative care setting to carry out research. Firstly, if I was to be attributed with an identity as some kind of expert, I did not think I could bring it off. Of course, I am familiar with aspects of hospice and palliative care but my own nursing experience is with patients with cancer. I have not worked in a specialised palliative care culture or hospice. I therefore consider myself an outsider within this context. Secondly, it may be thought that I was in some sense overly inquisitive and/or attempting to evaluate the work going on in such settings. To combat the potential for these concerns surfacing, I did emotion work on myself so as to appear relaxed and agreeable, friendly and informal. My goal was to enable all levels of staff to feel comfortable when I was around. I decided to carry off the research role by working at a demeanour of approachability, and to push the help I needed from the staff to accomplish the research. Coffey and Atkinson (1996) say that one cannot control how others perceive your participation. I agree with this but I believe you can manage it. My impression management was to hold an outward demeanour of being friendly, watching and listening carefully, greeting people, and using good eye contact. I decided not to ask too many questions, as this in itself might be perceived as threatening to some people. This self-management did shape the data and meant that I would avoid asking too many questions unless invited to do so. I worked at my non-verbal behaviour and attempted to look engaged, animated, alert and interested in everything that was going on. This enabled a degree of acceptability and to be hopefully seen as non-threatening.

I wondered what social category the group would assign to me. I decided when explaining my research that I would emphasise the fact that I was a part-time research student while working as a lecturer. I felt that if I was perceived as an expert, this would not help me as I was not an expert in hospice work. Of course, I did not want to be positioned as a critic. This would mean that people might be defensive with me or might avoid me. I monitored this by paying attention to emotions, for example, how I was greeted and non-verbal behaviour towards me. The social worker left a note for me and the title she gave me was 'research nurse'. The nurses were concerned about who I was rather than what I wanted. For example, the team leaders quickly found out about where I lived and my family situation, and this helped to reduce feelings of social distance. I felt that the team leaders were going to help me and were not going to put obstacles in my way. In this context, my social and family circumstances matched my hosts' and this enabled me to present myself in a non-threatening way with the nurses. The ethnographer should create different self-presentations for different settings according to Walsh (2004). This identifies the dynamic nature of presenting oneself, which required emotion work and interpersonal skills.

I found that one of the most tiring aspects of being an ethnographer and the emotion work needed was finding a balance between the different roles one has to play. I found that being constantly alert to how one is being positioned by the practitioners in the field as well as positioning oneself to get the best out of the situation as emotionally tiring. For example, I always arrived at the hospice a little early so that I could get mentally prepared and psyched up for whatever would be required of me to access data. Indeed, Li (2002) explores the distressing situation when her fieldwork was almost scuppered by a hostile member of the nursing staff. At this time, Li experienced the emotional reaction of 'loathing and the desire to withdraw' described by Lofland and Lofland (1984). She managed to stay in the field and complete her fieldwork by getting good support within her research and supervisory network.

Fortunately for her she found a sympathetic sponsor within the hospice team despite the resistance of one of the nurses. Many writers agree that in all stages of the ethnographic enterprise, social relationships remain key (Coffey, 1999; Hammersley & Atkinson, 1995; Walsh, 2004). I found that keeping on good terms with people, avoiding looking strained or irritable requires a degree of thought and emotion management—similar I suspect to acting or going onstage (Goffman, 1959). However, although social relationships need to be smoothed and negotiated as access to data often depends on these relationships, rich data can also be acquired through being reflective when encountering resistance. Persistence can pay off even in hostile territory if one has the time to be patient and to get good support during the process (Lawton, 2000; Li, 2002).

Observer as Participant

I prepared to take on the role of observer as participant within the hospice setting. This role achieves a balance in favour of observation over participation (Junker, 1960). According to Junker, most overt ethnography takes up a position between the observer as participant and participant as observer roles. Most writers agree that the marginal positioning is the best place to be (Junker, 1960; Hammersley & Atkinson, 1995). However, this can be difficult and can cause some emotional strain in keeping this positioning. For example, Frank (2004) says it can be difficult to keep your balance on a boundary in that we can fall back in to ourselves or forward into the other. This experience of falling in to the 'other' was experienced by Rager (2005) who describes how she cried together with her respondents during her research involving women with breast cancer. Thus, within a relationship, one needs an acceptable level of distance and difference so that there is a space between two people to enable dialogue, according to Frank. Lofland and Lofland (1984) produce a typology of different sources of emotional stress caused by fieldwork. This includes: deception and fear of disclosure, loathing and the desire to withdraw, sympathy and the impulse to help, marginality and the 'temptation to convert'. For my own work, the latter two points are important. In the next section, I will discuss the 'temptation to convert' to the complete participant, sometimes referred to as 'going native', and the pull back to being an observer. I will discuss this tension in relation to a visit with one of the community palliative care nurses.

'Temptation to Convert'

I visited a patient with one of the community palliative care nurses. This was going to be a difficult visit as the district nurse had alerted the community palliative care nurse to a problematic situation connected to the patient. The patient's husband was reported to have touched the district nurse inappropriately and Rachel, the community palliative care nurse, was anxious about this. This is what I recorded in my research journal:

1 What is all the fuss about? The patient's husband has had a stroke and sometimes
2 this sort of behaviour can occur. Why is Rachel so edgy about the visit? Perhaps it
3 is because she is in the late stages of pregnancy. She is glad I am accompanying
4 her on this visit. Perhaps I should be worried, there may be a 'scene' in the house
5 and perhaps Rachel may become upset.
Extract from research journal
6 We visited Eileen today she looked slight, quiet, frail and worried I thought. I
7 wondered what exactly had gone on with the district nurse? Eileen's daughter was
8 with her and she was very welcoming and friendly. There was no sign of the
9 husband. As we entered the house I felt very alert and I surveyed the room and
10 Rachel settled herself in an armchair near Eileen. Then I found somewhere to sit
11 facing the door so I could see anyone entering the room and to my left there was
12 access to the kitchen. I was making a mental note of all the exits from the room
13 and I found myself rehearsing what to do should the husband appear and do

14 something that upset Rachel and the family. Rachel started her assessment and I
15 felt very alert and watchful. Rachel asked 'where is your husband?' and Eileen said
16 he was upstairs as 'he gets up quite late'. I wondered if he had been told to stay
17 upstairs until we had gone. After about one hour, I could hear the patient's husband
18 moving about upstairs. I thought 'oh no he is going to come downstairs now just
19 as we are about to leave'. I couldn't wait to get out of the house. But I kept what
20 I hoped was a 'cool demeanour'.

Extract from research journal

When we visited the patient I suddenly found myself in a situation where I might have to take some action as I thought there might be a scene in the house (line 4). I also was aware that Rachel was pleased I was accompanying her on the visit; perhaps then I had a part to play (line 3, 4). I found I was worrying about physical and spatial safety by making notes of all the exits and entrances from the room (line 12). I was rehearsing how to do emotion work managing my own emotions (line 10) to prepare to save face for the family and for Rachel, should an incident occur (Goffman, 1959; Hochschild, 1983). I was therefore completely involved in this situation, thinking as a practitioner would: planning where to sit to get a good view of the room (line 11), making mental notes (line 12) and rehearsing in my mind what to do (line 13). I enjoyed the feeling of complete involvement and the fact that I had a part to play. I suppose I felt useful. Gerrish (2003), a researcher and also a trained nurse, describes how she felt vulnerable when she visited a young woman with terminal breast cancer with the district nurse. She felt the district nurse was using her as a colleague, someone who could listen to the district nurse's concerns and a sense of reciprocity developed. Unlike Gerrish, I did not feel vulnerable but I did experience the sense of reciprocity with Rachel. Rather than being an observer, I was completely involved in this situation and I, like, Rachel was worried (line 18).

Having written down what happened in my research diary I forgot about this incident until it was discussed later at the palliative care team meeting. At the palliative care team meeting I was asked a direct question about the visit:

Nurse R: But when I was asking about the husband, I wanted to know how he was two years ago, before the stroke, you know, because and they were very hesitant about coming forward with that weren't they?
AA: Mm. Mm
Nurse R: We didn't get, what I expected them to say was oh he was a lovely man. He was a lovely dad and it is such a shame. We didn't get any of that. She just looked down. So, you know, I'm not sure and apparently he's got a CPN as well and he goes to Charles wing to day-care because when he went to a normal day care he kept fondling everybody, he was, they put him in Charles Wing
(Laughter)

Audio recording of palliative care team meeting

Rachel sought my opinion about the visit at line 3: 'they were very hesitant about coming forward with that weren't they?' I could not frame a reply that I thought would be satisfactory; in effect I went blank. This was uncomfortable for me and I felt tense. I got over the incident by encouraging Rachel to continue to tell the story herself by my response 'Mm Mm' (line 4). I felt I was letting Rachel down by not being able to construct a reply that would sound articulate and meet the expectation of the team. Rachel uses 'we' twice at lines 5 and 6. I believe that in this talk Rachel is positioning me as a member of the team, a colleague through her use of '*we* didn't get' (line 5) and again '*we* didn't get any of that' (line 6). Together 'we' observed and experienced what is reported by Rachel and furthermore this was discussed between us in the car on the way back to the hospice. However, by not being able to reply in a satisfactory manner I felt similar to that described by actors as 'corpsing'. I was completely frozen and unable to respond in an appropriate manner. I now understood 'the fear of disclosure' identified by Lofland and Lofland (1984). I was not playing my part as an insider properly, not being able to offer a fluent reply and I thought this was being displayed in the meeting.

As the talk went on, it became more humorous and in the next excerpt of data there is laughter at my reported reaction to the incident, which relieved the tension I was feeling:

1 Nurse R: He's does most of the time when he goes. I mean apparently he doesn't like it. He
2 kicks up a bit of a stink about it but most of the time he goes. So I think probably your safest
3 to ring. Make sure he's gone. He was upstairs when we were there (laughing). Anne had a
4 quick getaway in the kitchen didn't you? She worked it all out. We were all right. So it was
5 okay. But it was a bit very intimidating for carers and of course for her.

Audio recording of palliative care team meeting

The story was told with some humour and there was laughter about the situation and my reported reaction to this situation: '*She* worked it all out. *We* were all right' (line 4). In this utterance, I am being presented as someone who 'worked it out' so Rachel is presenting me as competent in the situation. I also had not been able to tell Rachel who was in the late stages of pregnancy that I was worried about her safety and the 'quick getaway in the kitchen' (line 4) was a strategy for me to be mobile and allow me to intervene if needed. This incident in the team meeting made clear to me the tension of being in a marginal place balancing involvement with detachment, and I think this is what caused the feeling of discomfort. I did not think I could maintain objectivity if I started to take on a status as a type of insider. A researcher who cannot stand back from the knowledge they have acquired may face analytic problems (Coffey, 1999). I had not planned on being part of the action but clearly in this situation it was difficult to control. Participant observation is referred to as an 'oscillating situation' (Kirk & Miller, 1986, p. 7). The oscillating uncertainty on this occasion was around, which identity was going to be given, or withheld and the fact that I had to react in an appropriate manner; for example, thinking as a practitioner in terms of safety and a researcher in terms of the data. The tension that this situation engendered was similar to the identity crisis discussed by Jarvie (1969). He says it is not possible to be both a stranger and a friend, and the identity crisis that may arise precipitates an integrity crisis and one role overrides the other to resolve the crisis. Thus, temporarily, the professional practitioner role overrides the research role during the community visit.

Listening to data or reading transcripts of data means that the intensity of the fieldwork experiences are relived time and time again. Emotion work is required at this time when listening and re-listening to interviews of sensitive and sometimes upsetting material, which can unsettle the researcher especially when starting out in their research career (Malacrida, 2007). When transcribing data, the intensity of the experience was relived and reflected on. I asked myself: what does the ethnographer's experience mean for the data? This question took some time to answer, but it became a key analytic category for my research and I found what doing reputation was about for me the researcher as well as for my research participants (Arber, 2004). This was an important analytic category for my data analysis. Listening to audios of the data and reading transcripts when coding brings the researcher back to the experience and therefore the experiences in the field are relived.

Ethnography is often conducted by members of a culture or related cultures rather than by complete strangers and these cultures are not homogenous (Coffey, 1999). So according to Coffey, one can interrogate what is a stranger or a member, or an outsider or an insider. She continues that a *self* is crafted through personal relationships and interactions between the researcher and those that are researched. Thus, the issue of identity is not fixed but malleable. Role and identity can therefore be defined and redefined by oneself and by others, and this is what can cause discomforting feelings when expectations about identity are not shared at any given moment. Similarly, Stanworth (2004) describes how her status as a researcher was transformed into confidante, confessor, comforter and judge when researching the sources of meaning of people who are dying. This malleability and fluidity of identities given and taken is perhaps characteristic of all relationships. However, such identities and roles can also constrain. I did feel uncomfortable when observing distressed patients and relatives. For example, one day the doctor had some sad news for the relatives of a very sick patient. The relatives broke down crying. I felt caught in a dilemma and asked myself: 'What should I do? Should I try and offer some comfort to the relatives as a nurse would do?'

I was aware that there was no nurse present. The tension between being a researcher and a nurse was strong but on this occasion, I kept the researcher boundary in place even though I felt very uncomfortable about this. I used my fieldwork journal to reflect on this experience. I note in my research journal, 'one of the most distressing aspects of observing distress is not being able to have an active role in relation to this'. By this I mean that a nurse would have a part to play in consoling and comforting the relatives but a researcher can only witness the distress and write about it. For the researcher to become a nurse on this occasion I felt may cause some embarrassment for the team. Conversely it may have not been a problem for the team at all but a judgement I had made and a boundary I had put in place.

Enabling Reflexivity

One of the ways of enabling reflexivity is by keeping a journal. Keeping journals as distinct from field notes enables one to keep track of theoretical perspectives and assumptions as well as keep track of emotional reactions (Gilbert, 2001). According to Lofland (1971, p. 234), keeping a journal is not only for recording the setting but 'for 'recording' the observer as well'. Most researchers and writers agree with this, and keeping a journal may enable understanding through self-reflection and avoid a tendency to self-absorption (Kleinman & Copp, 1993; Rosaldo, 1989). Thus, closeness and distance is not only about experiences and reflections on the field but also about how one feels and the emotions that may be engendered. Recording of personal opinions, emotions, and responses to being an observer according to Lofland (1971) enables the observer to keep track of such events, which may be useful later during analysis. This is a particular issue for those studying members of a group to which they have membership or professional affiliation (Edwards, 2002) such as clinicians, therapists and nurses as they have to negotiate a research relationship rather than a therapeutic relationship. Furthermore, the therapist or nurse may feel a tension between the role of nurse or therapist and researcher (Arber, 2004; Gilbert, 2001).

I completed a fieldwork diary every time I went in to the research setting. I also planned to give a conference paper on my fieldwork experience (Arber, 2001). At this conference, another researcher talked about his experience of ethnographic fieldwork describing how he felt scared to go into the acute psychiatric ward due to the threatening behaviour of a couple of patients (Quirk, 2001). He expressed the same feeling that I had about getting psyched up to go into the research situation, but unlike Quirk I did not have a feeling of being scared but more a feeling of apprehension. The feeling of isolation that could arise during fieldwork was balanced by belonging to a social network of research students with time spent socialising and discussing research informally (Wincup, 2001). Other strategies suggested for dealing with the emotions engendered by research include counselling, peer debriefing/review, 'creating space' and relaxation techniques (Edwards, 2002; Rager, 2005). In fact, Rager recommends that preparation for researchers should include information on appropriate self-care strategies to avoid 'compassion stress'.

Credibility and Reliability

The types of 'self' that are presented within research may enable claims about authenticity such as 'being there' and to enable the reader to judge the validity of the whole enterprise by being transparent about the 'goings on' in the field (Seale, 1999; The AM, 2002). Credibility and reliability can be improved by firstly identifying the particular status position taken by the researcher, as this sheds light on what can and cannot be observed. For example, Li (2002) was unable to observe 'critical moments' as staff indicated her presence in the patient's room was not welcome. Therefore, some of the data she presents reflects her role as an outsider. As Lee (1993, p. 6) points out, the feelings engendered in researching sensitive topics such as death and dying mean that the researcher as well as the researched may have to share feelings 'of unease, discomfort or emotional pain'. These feelings may then affect what we are allowed and prepared to observe. Secondly, it is important to be reflective about who offered data and the context in which it was offered. Finally, there should be a full account of theories that informed the research (LeCompte & Goetz,

1982). These are all components of reflexivity and help the reader to assess the credibility of research findings according to Seale (1999). Part of an audit trail of the research process could include independent examination of entries in the researchers' journal or diary by the supervisor for example to identify daily activities, and sampling techniques (Lincoln & Guba, 1985; Seale, 1999). Documenting one's feelings and emotions about the identities and roles assumed and taken can also be a useful part of the audit trail. Participant observation is conscious work requiring the observer to understand the process of transformation which s/he undergoes, by being present in the field (Baszanger & Dodier, 1997). Thus, during the research journey the researcher describes in what capacity s/he was present and the place s/he occupied during fieldwork.

Strategies for Reflexivity in the Field

- Keep a research diary to document the researcher's feelings and emotions; this enables emotional reflexivity.
- Good support is essential for the researcher, including informal support such as that provided by one's colleagues and peer group.
- Supervisors should be knowledgeable about how to support students appropriately, for example listening to the student's experience, reading the fieldwork diary and encouraging regular supervision.
- Self-care strategies such as 'time out', relaxation techniques, debriefing and counselling strategies should be carefully considered before, during and after fieldwork, as experiences such as those described have implications for emotional well-being.

Conclusion

The experience of being an outsider, an insider and on the boundary between these two roles can cause some strain for the researcher. I have reflected on some moments where I experienced being an insider and an outsider and the self-management involved to maintain my footing as a researcher and sometimes unexpectedly as a practitioner. The 'temptation to convert' is discussed as a seductive option as this allows a feeling of homeostasis across the insider outsider boundary, which enables the researcher to be 'at home' in the practitioner role. Yet having an identity as an insider allows access to data that may not be accessed by an outsider. In conclusion, the ethnographer needs a level of preparedness for undertaking demanding fieldwork in the context of healthcare whether they have a practitioner/therapist background or not. A reflexive approach enables one to understand how the researcher who is also a practitioner has an impact on those researched. It also means that a researcher with such a background should interrogate their own beliefs and feelings in the same way that they interrogate those of others. Thus, at all stages in the research the impact of the researcher in terms of access to data, relationships in the field, and how one is addressed as a researcher, as a practitioner or both should be documented and become part of one's analysis.

This chapter is based on a paper published in the Journal of Nursing Research in 2006 and is reproduced and updated for this book with permission from the publishers.

References

Arber, A. (2001). Getting in and staying in: Negotiating and maintaining access to a hospice setting. *Ethnography and Health Care Conference*, Royal College of Nursing, London, Saturday, 8 December 2001.

Arber, A. (2004). Building reputation: The significance of pain talk in hospice and palliative care team meetings. PhD thesis, Goldsmiths College, University of London.

Back, L. (2002). Dancing and wrestling with scholarship: Things to do and things to avoid in a PhD Career. *Sociological Research Online, 7*, 4. Retrieved November 30, 2002, from www.socresonline.org.uk/7/4/back.html

Baszanger, I., & Dodier, N. (1997). Ethnography relating parts to the whole. In D. Silverman (Ed.), *Qualitative research* (pp. 8–23). London: Sage.

Brewer, J. D. (1994). The ethnographic critique of ethnography. In C. Seale (Ed.), *Social research methods a reader* (pp. 405–411). London: Routledge.

Charmaz, K. (2004). Premises, principles, and practices in qualitative research: Revisiting the foundations. *Qualitative Health Research, 14*(7), 976–993.

Coffey, A. (1999). *The ethnographic self.* London: Sage.

Coffey, A., & Atkinson, P. (1996). *Making sense of qualitative data*. London: Sage.

Edwards, B. (2002). Deep insider research. *Qualitative Research Journal, 2*(1), 71–84.

Frank, A. (2004). *The renewal of generosity: Illness, medicine and how to live*. Chicago: University of Chicago Press.

Gerrish, K. (2003). Self and others: The rigour and ethics of insider ethnography. In J. Latimer (Ed.), *Advanced qualitative research for nursing* (pp. 77–94). Oxford: Blackwell.

Gilbert, K. R. (2001). Introduction: Why are we interested in emotions? In K. R. Gilbert (Ed.), *The emotional nature of qualitative research*. London: CRC Press.

Goffman, E. (1959). *The presentation of self in everyday life*. London: Penguin.

Gouldner, A. W. (1972). Towards a reflexive sociology. In C. Seale (Ed.), *Social research methods* (pp. 381–383). London: Routledge.

Gubrium, J., & Holstein, J. (1997). *The new language of qualitative method*. Buckingham: Open University Press.

Hammersley, M., & Atkinson, P. (1995). *Ethnography principles in practice* (2nd ed.). London: Routledge.

Hochschild, A. (1983). *The managed heart: The commercialisation of human feeling*. Berkley: University of California Press.

Jarvie, I. C. (1969). The problem of ethical integrity in participant observation. *Anthropology, 10*(5), 505–508.

Junker, B. (1960). *Field work*. Chicago: University of Chicago Press.

Kirk, J., & Miller, M. L. (1986). *Reliability and validity in qualitative research*. London: Sage.

Kleinman, S., & Copp, M. A. (1993). *Emotions and fieldwork*. London: Sage.

Lawton, J. (2000). *The dying process patients' experiences of palliative care*. London: Routledge.

LeCompte, M., & Goetz, J. (1982). Problems of reliability and validity in ethnographic research. *Review of Educational Research, 52*(1), 31–60.

Lee, R. M. (1993). *Doing research on sensitive topics*. London: Sage.

Li, S. (2002). Symbiotic niceness: A study of psychosocial care in palliative care settings. PhD thesis, Goldsmiths College, University of London.

Lincoln, Y. S., & Guba, E. (1985). *Naturalistic enquiry*. Beverly Hills: Sage.

Lofland, J. (1971). *Analyzing social settings: A guide to qualitative observation and analysis*. Belmont, CA: Wadsworth.

Lofland, J., & Lofland, L. H. (1984). *Analyzing social settings: A guide to qualitative observation and analysis*. Belmont, CA: Wadsworth.

Malacrida, C. (2007). Reflexive journaling on emotional research topics: Ethical issues for team researchers. *Qualitative Health Research, 17*(10), 1329–1339.
Miller, J., & Glassner, B. (2004). The "inside" and the "outside". Finding realities in interviews. In D. Silverman (Ed.), *Qualitative research: Theory, method and practice* (pp. 51–66). London: Sage.
Pollner, M. (1987). *Mundane reason*. New York: Cambridge University Press.
Quirk A (2001) Anxiety in ethnography: Studying life on acute psychiatric wards. *Ethnography and Health Care Conference*, Royal College of Nursing, Cavendish Square, London, Saturday, 8 December 2001.
Rager, K. B. (2005). Compassion stress and the qualitative researcher. *Qualitative Health Research, 15*(3), 423–430.
Rosaldo, R. (1989). *Culture and truth: The remaking of social analysis*. London: Routledge.
Seale, C. (1998). *Researching society and culture*. London: Sage.
Seale, C. (1999). *The quality of qualitative research*. London: Sage.
Silverman, D. (2001). *Interpreting qualitative data methods for analyzing talk, text and interaction* (2nd ed.). London: Sage.
Stanworth, R. (2004). *Recognising spiritual needs in people who are dying*. Oxford: Oxford University Press.
The AM. (2002). *Palliative care and communication: Experiences in the clinic*. Buckingham: Open University Press.
Walsh, D. (2004). Doing ethnography. In C. Seale (Ed.), *Researching society and culture* (pp. 225–238). London: Sage.
Wincup, E. (2001). Feminist research with women awaiting trial: The effects on participants in the qualitative research process. In K. R. Gilbert (Ed.), *The emotional nature of qualitative research* (pp. 17–35). London: CRC Press.

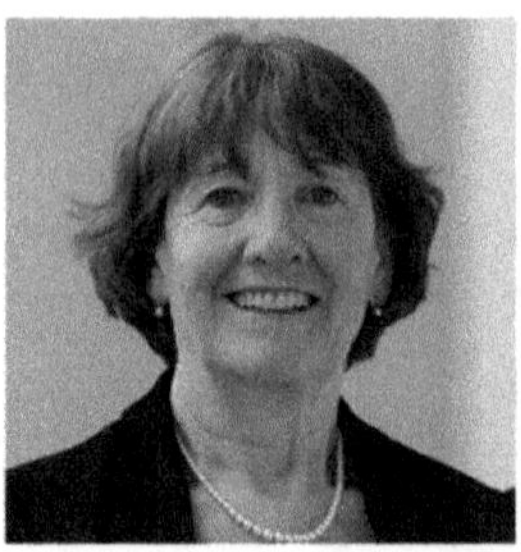

Anne Arber is Senior Lecturer in Cancer and Palliative Care, School of Health Sciences, University of Surrey, Guildford, Surrey, UK. Anne was awarded her Ph.D. in 2004 from Goldsmiths, University of London, UK. Anne conducts research in cancer and palliative care. She has supervised Ph.D. and clinical doctorate students since 2004.

5

Ethics and Reflexivity in Researching HIV-Related Infertility

Tam Chipawe Cane

Introduction

In this chapter, I draw on fieldwork conducted for my doctorate that explored the lived experiences of people living with HIV (PLWHIV). I was interested in PLWHIV who had accessed fertility treatment and child adoption services. HIV-related infertility and adoption are different to other forms of infertility or experiences of adoption because some of those affected may not be biologically infertile. When untreated, HIV can affect reproduction and increase the risk of HIV transmission during unprotected sexual intercourse to both a non-positive partner and potentially an unborn baby. Consequently, PLWHIV who wish to become parents are generally encouraged to access counselling in order to establish safer methods of having children. Fertility treatment or adoption are possible options that avoid the risk of HIV transmission to the unborn baby and partner (Savasi, Mandia, Laoreti & Certin, 2013). In this chapter, I

T.C. Cane (✉)
Department of Psychology, Social Work and Counselling, University of Greenwich, London, UK

H.T. Allan, A. Arber (eds.), *Emotions and reflexivity in Health and Social Care Field Research*, https://doi.org/10.1007/978-3-319-65503-1_5

discuss how I managed professional and personal relationships during fieldwork as I researched a small community of PLWHIV.

I was interested in the subjective experiences of PLWHIV and their inner life-worlds as they sought fertility treatment and/or adoption. I used Interpretive Phenomenological Analysis (IPA) as my methodological framework to achieve a reflexive stance during my research. I thought that bracketing my emotions and previous experiences was impractical. This was because I was a practising social worker who sometimes engaged with this client group. I found it crucial to find ways to maintain boundaries during the research process so that I could be in a safe place to do my research. I spent time reflecting on my previous knowledge, practice experiences and conceptions using a process called internal dialogue (Maccarini & Prandini, 2010). I had internal dialogues with myself about the sensitivity of the data, and about what was potentially going to be shared with me. A typical dialogue went something like this: 'I am entrusted with information that has not been shared with others, can I emotionally cope with this and is my approach potentially harmful?' This internal dialogue enabled me to think about my capacities, ethics and boundaries as I knew my study was going to be emotionally challenging.

Many of the emotions I experienced were completely unanticipated and resulted from the participants sharing their experiences of secrecy and stigma in relation to adoption and/or fertility treatment. Their emotions raised profound feelings in me which I needed to reflect upon. As a consequence, I found that subjectivity *and* intersubjectivity were strong dynamics in the research between me and the participants. Since qualitative research involves dyadic interactions between people, reflexivity requires an interplay between the researcher and the participants' subjective worlds of experience, giving rise to intersubjective dynamics and understanding (Finlay, 2002). I used reflexivity as an active internal dialogue about a complicated situation (Maccarini & Prandini, 2010).

I developed my internal dialogue as a process of self-examination involving scrutiny and understanding of any assumptions and biases that could affect the interpretation of participants' experiences. This included looking into my personal opinions, feelings, emotions to understand how they were employed during the research alongside the interpretation of stories participants told me. For Wiley (2010), reflexive dialogues require researchers to see themselves as 'three legged stools, standing simultaneously in the past, present and the future' (2010, p. 19). In my internal dialogues, I reflected on my *past* self by exploring professional and personal experiences brought to the research, the knowledge and existing emotions associated with the emotive interviews (the *present*) and the analysis of the data, which offered me the opportunity to manage my emotions without causing harm to participants and self in order to formulate a better understanding of participants' life-worlds as they sought to move forward (the *future*). In addition, as part of an action-orientated research approach, Wiley supposes that reflexivity requires imagination about future actions and their consequences whilst, at the same time, engaging with the I (present self), the me (past self) and the you (future or critical self), all of which depend on the purpose, and the projected and anticipated actions as part of the research. For example, the past self was myself as a researcher who is also social worker, to which was added the experience of working with PLWHIV who have lost the ability to achieve biological conception. Therefore, the sense of loss was an awareness I had through my professional role as a social worker but was also a constant presence in the research interviews—the *I* in the present. The participant's future included hope that PLWHIV would adopt a child or bear children through fertility treatment—future self. In that respect, reflecting beyond the wider features presented during data collection facilitated a deeper understanding of the impact of unique narrative accounts on participants' lives.

I recruited participants through charitable organisations that support PLWHIV. An online recruitment hub was created to promote and facilitate recruitment. Where appropriate, I visited support group sessions to talk about my research as well as using magazines and leaflets. Most interviews took place at the research hub (an HIV charitable organisation that offered me an honorary research contract) where I had a dedicated room and support staff available if required. One interview was conducted in the participant's home for their convenience. Wherever the location of the interviews, I re-visited the risk assessment strategy I had devised: to observe participant responses, monitor the emotional impact of the research questions and review participants' safety as well as my own (Holmes, 2010). Observations associated with emotional presentation of participants during interviews were noted in a research log and they formed part of the analysis.

All the participants in the study were committed to having their children through fertility treatment or adoption. Some had accessed adoption after a series of failed reproductive treatments, whilst others had only opted for adoption. Some participants had successfully adopted children, others were unsuccessful or in the process of re-applying to adopt through a separate agency. Given the intrusive, demanding and sensitive nature of both fertility treatment and adoption investigations, some participants were traumatised and challenged psychologically (Carroll, 2012). Participants felt that the reasons for failed adoption may be due to negative social work assessments and discrimination. In addition, even when accessed, fertility treatments are expensive and largely unsuccessful. Both fertility treatment and adoption have the potential to trigger feelings of anxiety and distress, and the assessments associated with both these processes may appear unsupportive. Childlessness itself had been a problem for the participants, who experienced stigma, and cultural and/or social pressures. Additionally, HIV-related childlessness had caused devastation, sorrow, segregation, guilt and sometimes powerlessness and frustration. During the interviews, participants described feeling emotionally fragile because the processes of applying for and undergoing fertility treatment and adoption were challenging. Those procedures frequently reminded them of how HIV contributed to their 'infertility' or childlessness. Some participants relived their experiences of how they contracted HIV and how this affected their ability or chance to have children using natural methods to avoid the risk of transmitting HIV.

Because of their emotional state during the interviews, rapport building was important in order to foster relationships with the participants so they felt comfortable with me and the interview environment. Thus, preparatory empathy created a gateway for participants to willingly talk about their experiences. I found that participants sometimes spoke about experiences they had not shared with others due to the fear of stigma. Consequently, when participants felt distressed, the rapport that had been built allowed participants to feel comfortable enough to elaborate on their feelings. Personally, I chose not to disclose my feelings in order to facilitate the researcher relationship. I wanted participants to talk about their experiences without worrying about my emotions. I wanted them to appreciate that their story was recognised within the research relationship and that my research was a way of doing something about it. My aim was to go beyond text but towards deeper interpretative psychological and psychoanalytic interests (Smith, 2008).

Subsequent sections in this chapter will explore the importance of engaging in pre-fieldwork reflexive activities, the conflicts that may arise between the research role against other responsibilities, such as being a practioner. Strategies to mange reflexivity are proposed before closing the chapter.

Pre-reflective Activities

Processes of self-evaluation are subject to the researcher's philosophical position and the theoretical framework that grounds the research. During self-evaluation, I acknowledged how my involvement and relationship with the phenomenon I was studying could be enmeshed with past experiences. I completed pre-reflective activities before the research commenced by taking an inventory of my experiences, beliefs and values, and experiences (Archer, 2012; Finlay, 2002) and then before each interview. I found this useful prior to interviewing participants even where they had provided a brief outline of their story during the recruitment phase. As a social worker who had supported service users through HIV-related difficulties, I carried my own perceptions and views regarding the subject. Prior to that, during my social work training, I had supported and advised PLWHIV on how and where to access fertility treatment and adoption services. Even then, I identified discrimination and problems faced by PLWHIV when seeking parenthood through fertility services. My choice and experience of research with PLWHIV was influenced by my professional experience. Awareness of my pre-existing knowledge, of how I was co-constituted and situated within the methodology helped me to unravel subjective and a priori assumptions. I examined my position during and after each interview in order to identify intersubjectivities that deepened the interpretations of the subject under investigation (Finlay, 2002; Holmes, 2010).

As a researcher, I had no lived experience of HIV and HIV-related infertility, nor had I gone through HIV-related fertility treatment or child adoption procedures but I had social work experience in matters around HIV. For this reason, reflexivity was an important element for being aware of what I brought to the research in order to become an introspective tool for the research process (Finlay, 2002). I went through a difficult process of shifting my positioning from practitioner to researcher, which required acknowledging the ethical and power differences between the different roles. To achieve this, I consciously detached my social work role from the research process. This meant relocating myself as a researcher at the heart of the research. On the other hand, I could not completely replace my prior experience as a social worker however hard I tried to achieve this. For example, as a social worker I had been an advocate to empower service users, to educate, support and represent those seeking to adopt children by helping them to navigate through various stages of an adoption process. As a *researcher* undertaking research in my own area of practice, I was more concerned with listening to participants' stories. I avoided being an advocate, educator, assessor or advisor at the same time as being a researcher. I also consciously avoided using my professional knowledge. Professional knowledge can be a way of gaining power over participants. Social workers are often seen as figures of power and authority when making professional judgements (Ruch & Julkunen, 2016) and when they make decisions about the suitability of prospective adopter's ability to adopt. I avoided this by bracketing my professional knowledge through maintaining a research log and taking down accounts of various challenges throughout the process.

Reflexivity is a process that requires researchers to acknowledge their social interactions, use of language and shared meaning, and in so doing create intersubjective dialogues and dynamics between the researcher and participant in order to produce research knowledge (Maccarini & Prandini, 2010; Noble & Mcilveen, 2012). Reflexivity may also be an inward examination of thoughts, feelings and the use of one's body as an object in the experience of others (Crossley, 2006). For Crossley (2006), this requires engaging in silences and in self-policing whilst consciously acknowledging their own embodied, tacit and practice knowledge. The researcher may mirror the participant's experiences and their emotional responses, responding by internally deploying conscious emotional responses to what the participant is reporting.

Emotions and Disclosure in the Research Space

It was imperative for me to acknowledge my own 'humanness', to examine my own emotions and behaviours within the research environment (Finlay, 2002; Holmes, 2010). This helped me to monitor my reactions and to be appropriate in my conduct in an endeavour to not influence the participants' reactions (Sandelowski & Barroso, 2002). I managed the intensity of emotions occurring in each interview by remaining emotionally and physically calm to avoid causing distress to the participant. For me, a sense of uneasiness about upsetting participants was always present. Part of me hoped, at a certain level, that participants would not revisit the circumstances through which they contracted HIV. I was unsure of how I would deal with this. I also did not wish to cause harm to people by getting them to relive how they became HIV positive. I knew some of the stories were likely to be distressing. Perhaps my reluctance was recognised by some participants who made efforts to avoid causing me upset when they spoke about their life experiences. One male participant in a same-sex relationship spoke about how he contracted HIV; it was particularly stressing as his sexual partner had not shared his HIV positive status with him. This description was emotionally challenging for me. It is possible that he observed my efforts to contain my feelings at that time and he questioned:

> How will you deal with what I told you if you do not talk to someone you trust about this? I understand you have to keep what I told you confidential but I also understand if you talk to someone about it as long as you do not reveal my identity. You do not have to respond to this but it is natural that we all share difficult experiences with others.

This conversation was powerful. I did not respond verbally or immediately. I realised that this participant empathised with my feelings and how I had responded emotionally to his devastating story. In an internal dialogue after the interview, I realised that in this situation that I did not know how to respond verbally as I felt lost for words and engulfed by the devastating story he had shared with me. Perhaps in the interview he could read my non-verbal language and was now reaching out to offer me support.

Smythe, Ironside, Sims, Swenson, and Spence (2008) highlight that interpretative work requires the researcher to explore that which remains unknown, by making it known. This includes understanding the meaning of silences, unspoken or concealed emotions and feelings. I suggest that in these silences, what remains unspoken is not only about the research participant but also intimately linked to the researcher. Understanding an individual's story requires curiosity. This involves asking the right questions to obtain new insights, acknowledging previous knowledge and sharing empathy (Smythe et al., 2008). I was aware that, without using open-ended questions or probing even when I sense emotion, I would not access the unknown. I rehearsed sensitive questioning and how to manage emotions or unexpected responses. This is what I have already noted as preparatory empathy. When I commenced fieldwork, I had already appreciated that fieldwork would involve maintaining a balance in my physical reactions to maintain a stable emotional posture. Thus, reflexivity for me required going beyond my intellectual ability, emotional intelligence and critical thinking about historical influences, economic and political influences (Spence, 2016) about HIV, adoption and fertility issues. It required me to journey alongside the participants' personal journeys and to see through their eyes the experiences as they were told to me. However, the true feelings and thoughts of the other are never fully known, as empathy is limited; the researcher is trying to understand an experience that they perhaps may never really fully understand.

In one interview, a participant told me that because I was not HIV positive, I had not experienced his 'life-journey', I would never truly understand what it meant for him to be homosexual, HIV positive, to desire to become an adoptive parent for a child with learning disabilities and be told (directly) 'you will not live long enough to parent a child'. This was a disturbing message and of course it was absolutely true. As a person, a researcher and a social worker, I would never be able to fully comprehend what it meant to experience this range of factors but I was nevertheless emotionally affected by the enormity of the distress. This particular situation raises the importance of preparing for complex conversations during interviews. Engaging in emotion work is also important to ensure that participants feel safe and comfortable to question the researcher's own understanding of the sensitive subjects under investigation because qualitative interviews are conversational.

Conflicts Between the Research Role and Practitioner Role

Participants in my study described their lived experiences and I was 'the other' who had limited awareness and knowledge of how I would feel about, and what it is like to live with, being infertile and looking to adopt a child as a result of HIV. The following is a data extract from my research log:

> Mercy is a forty-five-year-old, HIV-positive female. Mercy was desperate to have a child with her husband who was HIV-negative. Mercy's fallopian tubes were blocked and this prevented her from having biological children. She was in denial about her infertility but was comfortable with her HIV diagnosis. Her unsuccessful application for NHS fertility treatment funding led Mercy to feel desperate for answers to her infertility. She became keen to adopt but had also been unsuccessful. (Research log)

Mercy knew I was a social worker and she was eager for my assistance and support. It seemed that in a way she wanted me to be her advocate. Following the interview with Mercy, she rang me almost monthly, seeking help and support. Mercy already knew where to access fertility treatment and adoption services but she was stuck behind what she believed to be *barriers* of HIV-related discrimination that firstly, prevented her from applying for fertility treatment funding; then secondly, her adoption application being rejected. Mercy had also received reproductive counselling through an HIV charitable organisation. My dilemma was that I could not give further advice—I was not acting as a social worker or indeed an advisor, I was a researcher. I had to maintain professionalism and to avoid giving Mercy false hope. For me, this was a clear dilemma because I had to maintain my role as a researcher first and a social worker second. Yet I was a social worker first; this role was embedded within me before I commenced the research.

Mercy's desperate state saddened and troubled me. The reality of someone struggling to have a child and feeling unsupported and desperate led me to empathise with Mercy. The sadness was increased by her (or my) powerlessness and helplessness. In an internal dialogue recorded in my field diary, I asked myself: am I a researcher, am I a practitioner or a support worker/advocate? Through reflexivity, I tapped into my social work skills around managing emotions, preparatory empathy, creating a safe research space in order to contain emotions in the interview but at the same time to continue with the interview. Here, I am suggesting that emotional regulation is a transferable skill that is also embodied. The management of feelings cannot be eliminated from the research process when attempting to make sense of human experiences. This means that I had to acknowledge Mercy's challenges and direct her sensitively towards further interview questions. I struggled with the conflict between being a researcher and an advocate. I experienced a great desire to be helpful; I imagined Mercy as my own service user to whom I felt a sense of responsibility. However, I needed to be honest about my limitations within the research role. I was lucky that I had access to clinical supervision to discuss this situation.

Maintaining the boundary between practice and research fuelled a sense of guilt as I felt (as a researcher) that I was denying support and assistance to someone who needed it. I also felt angry towards the social workers mentioned in the interviews and towards the system which the participants clearly felt was discriminatory. Some participants were adamant that their experiences had been discriminatory. As I had previously worked with social workers with minimal understanding of HIV, even some who had expressed judgemental views about HIV and parenting, I was unsurprised that some participants felt they had been discriminated against by social workers. However, I was shocked and angry about the extent to which discrimination was perceived by my participants to be at the heart of unsuccessful fertility treatment funding or adoption applications. Surely the stringent adoption procedures were necessary not discriminatory? I struggled to reconcile these experiences by wondering if some practitioners do not see things from the perspective of PLWHIV. Maintaining the boundary between professional social worker and student researcher was a real challenge.

Further conflicts between my practitioner and researcher roles arose during fieldwork as I continued to work as a social worker whilst I was completing my doctorate. I had an almost constant internal dialogue going on as I reflected on my practice in the light of the data collection. On the one hand, listening to participants in interviews made me aware of the subjective experiences of PLWHIV when seeking to become parents through fertility services or adoption and how they feel stigmatised and discriminated against by social workers. On the other hand, my colleagues could not understand how PLWHIV could be permitted to access fertility services or adopt. I found myself exasperated by what appeared to be the ignorance and prejudice I observed in my colleagues. However slowly, repeated informal discussions with colleagues about the nature of adoption for non-traditional service users (those with health issues) helped me to understand the knowledge gaps among practitioners. This ongoing internal conversation and external conversations with colleagues allowed me to reflect on the interaction between data and practitioner experiences as part of the analysis, to better enter and experience the life-world of PLWHIV who felt marginalised by adoption and fertility services. Consequently, I was able to view the situation from two contradictory positions: the first as a service provider and the second from the perspective of the researched who had either positive or negative feelings about the adoption or fertility systems and services. As the research progressed, I was better able to understand the perspective of the participants through similar internal dialogues. These dialogues involved examining myself (the social worker and researcher) as a researcher whose role was to work with the perspectives and experiences of the participants, and make meaning of those experiences on a case-by-case basis. By so doing, I made an attempt to avoid using practice experience not through bracketing but through reflexivity on those experiences (Binder, Holgersen, & Moltu, 2012). I focused on the rich life-stories told to me by the participants.

The more I interviewed the participants and listened to their stories, the more I saw a system that was non-inclusive; this insight was challenging to work with. It is important for researchers to rely on their interpretative resources to formulate meaning. I struggled to 'exit the worlds of participants' in order to re-engage with my interpretative resources and to analyse and interpret the data. In particular, when I conducted textual interpretation, I became overly sensitive towards participants' experiences (Smith, 2012). Academic supervision, where I questioned data against my own practice experience, a priori assumptions and prejudices, helped me to recognise how I was situated in the interpretation process. Supervision therefore improved textual construction, that is, how to write without making my own assumptions beyond what is located in a given data extract (Davies, 2008). Extra care and attention was paid to each individual participant's transcript by consciously engaging in an active internal dialogue to facilitate a balanced analytical process (Maccarini & Prandini, 2010). Through interpretative activities, such as rough note-taking, writing, re-writing and supervisory support, this process became easier.

Ethical Dilemmas When Researching a Shared Community

While I did not interview those I had known before the research commenced, as a researcher with an African background, the potential for interviewing people from my own community was always a possibility. By the time I commenced fieldwork, I quickly realised that researching HIV in the UK brought me into contact with people from various African communities including my own. Holmes (2010) describes this as relationality. Conducting research in a community where I had social relations created an unexpected power dynamic, which threatened to interfere with my researcher position. A personal dilemma that occurred during fieldwork is illustrative of ethical dilemmas that may occur in research in a shared community.

> During my data collection phase, I arranged a focus group meeting with PLWHIV through a third sector agency. This was for the purpose of research briefing and recruitment (data collection where appropriate). The meeting was scheduled an hour before a peer to peer support group. After the first hour, peer to peer support focused on issues around HIV diagnosis and associated concerns. Prior to the first meeting commencing, all introductions, information and consent forms were completed. Three quarters of an hour after the first meeting, a relative of mine joined the group. In order to provide

> information, to seek consent and for introductions to take place, it was vital to pause group discussions and welcome Lorry accordingly. This was Lorry's first time in attending a support group. He attended on that day to seek support about his new diagnosis. Upon Lorry's request and the groups' agreement, group discussions were deviated in order to focus on Lorry, who presented a troubled situation. He was worried, anxious and desperate for support. The research discussions were terminated and the support group was directed accordingly by the HIV Coordinator who was present throughout.

I was able to reflect and consider the appropriateness of continuing with data collection in a space where a relation of mine found comfort, help and support. My internal dialogue led me to question whether or not I needed to engage in a personal conversation with Lorry or to completely disregard Lorry's presence. I began to feel uncomfortable about the power that I had acquired over Lorry through my new role as a researcher about his position as a PLWHIV and what effect this had on my role as a family member. I have already highlighted earlier the dilemma I faced over the dual roles I found myself in, but in this case, I had three roles—a social worker, a researcher and a relative. As in other situations, in this space I was there as a researcher, not as a friend or family member, or a support worker/group facilitator. Had Lorry arrived early he could have opted out or I could have foregone my research briefing session. I sensed, during the session, that neither Lorry nor I could escape. Given the sensitive nature of HIV, my internal dialogue is presented in the box below:

> I was concerned about Lorry worrying about his secret. Could Lorry trust that I would not disclose his secret? When he provided consent he was informed I was bound by confidentiality policies. However, I was not sure this would have been enough for him. In this case for me, reflexivity was not just an internal dialogue but negotiation of emotions that were physically sensed directly from Lorry. I could feel that physically, I was taking on Lorry's emotions and yet I was also managing my own emotions and my body language. Partly, I was shocked and overwhelmed by Lorry's story and his disclosures.

> Lorry's story was dramatic as he revealed how he had contracted HIV and how this affected his physical health at the time as well as the impact of the illness on his closest family, (in fact, he kept his HIV status from his wife and wider family). As I tuned into Lorry's story, I made a conscious decision to make no contributions to avoid eye contact show no facial responses but to remain silent. Although I did not ask him directly about his feelings but as I reflected after the interview, I wondered how Lorry felt about my silence. I wondered if Lorry felt a sense of reassurance when sharing his personal and social experiences in my presence. He could have inaccurately assumed that I shared the same 'status' (HIV positive) as him. I found myself working on reproducing my social presentation throughout this meeting by engaging in emotion work so that my conduct remained professional and appropriate.

Holmes (2010) states that understanding the social self and reproducing the self requires paying attention to one's emotions through a reflexive process. For this reason, the generalised other played a part in how I made decisions to remain in the room, contain my emotions, kept silent and managed my physical reactions. I did this by asking: how would Lorry and the other group members feel? How would others view me? What would the group say about me and my conduct and how would this look professionally? In this dialogue, I was concerned about my reputation with the group members and how my behaviour would be scrutinised and observed.

Research can be complex. Without understanding one's position in fieldwork and in the interpretation of data, the researcher may misrepresent the stories told and create a false impression when research environments become messy, as in the situation with Lorry. I had to make a judgement about whether recruiting from such a complex group environment was appropriate. I concluded that using HIV support groups to recruit participants was no longer viable. I concluded that ethical codes for research and practice need to be flexible enough to address the difficult feelings that arise in the field. Codes of conduct that promoted reflexivity and patient safety (Haggerty, 2004) were key to addressing the dilemmas HIV researchers face (Skovdal & Abebe, 2012).

As data collection progressed, it became clear that I, as the researcher, needed support. Immediately after the group session related above, I was left with emotions that I could not process at that time of the night (9 pm). I felt constrained by confidentiality policies, as I could not seek support from close friends or family although eventually I was able to speak to a research buddy without breaking confidentiality. Writing about my feelings, observations and experience in my reflexive log helped me to manage some of my feelings. Writing a reflective summary about the group session above and how it had gone helped me to reflect and revisit methodological perspectives of my research. In an ideal world, immediate supervision with buddies and research supervisors who are bound to the research codes of practice will help the researcher to process immediate feelings and emotions that arise during fieldwork.

Learning from Managing Strong Emotions

Conducting HIV-related research required a strong capability in respect to emotional containment and resilience. I found that I had to manage my own feelings and remain professional even when I heard distressing stories. When preparing for research, I was ready to engage as the instrument for data collection and data analysis. I had pre-reflected on how to react when witnessing others' emotions using preparatory empathy. I would argue that this is more than personal introspection (Finlay, 2002), which involves internal searching (Archer, 2010). Despite my preparations, I had not imagined the intensity of my own emotions. My practitioner experience as a social worker and my previous work with PLWHIV as an HIV support coordinator was insufficient in preparing me for dealing with the uncertain and unpredictable stories that the participants told. I felt both angry and sad after the interviews. My research buddies were often helpful to me in managing my own feelings. Although supervision was also helpful, this was not always scheduled at the times that I needed support.

One example of an interview that was particularly emotional, which I found upsetting and disturbing, was with a serodiscordant couple whose partner had HIV and haemophilia. He was desperate to receive fertility treatment funding through the National Health Service and distraught about his condition. He just wanted the NHS to at least fund all their reproductive treatment cycles, but without success. The couple used all their savings and eventually gave up. They were turned down by a number of adoption agencies. They put this down to HIV-related prejudice. Listening to their moving story, I physically felt the pain and anger on their behalf:

> I felt, no matter how middle class you are, no matter how qualified and what your social status is, HIV has the potential to ruin a loving couple's desire for (biological) parenthood. Systemic procedures and practitioner knowledge in fact, does not cater for people's back-stories and their desperation. Whatever they tried, they reached a 'brick-wall'. I respected the couple for challenging discrimination and remaining solid in their fight for parenthood. In my powerless position, I wondered, does it take a change in attitude for practitioners to realise that HIV does not always affect one's ability to bring up a child. After all, this couple is living well. They have now successfully adopted two children. It took only one agency and one practitioner with an open mind and open attitude to HIV. Did they have to fight through a plethora of agencies and fight against what they saw as discriminatory objections as much as they did? (Research log)

I was angry at how oppressive my participants found the systems they had to work with. One way of managing this was to use these feelings as clues for exploring the participants' experience further. Whilst it was appropriate to become attuned with participants' emotions, I was worried about my own feelings contaminating the pureness of the story as it was told and experienced by the participant. On the other hand, I needed to examine the meaning attached to their experiences and acknowledge why I had felt emotionally burdened by it. It was not about me but the experience of the participants. So, numbing my feelings, withholding comments, listening actively involved using emotion work but enabled me to access participant stories by asking probing questions to understand the meaning they had placed on their experiences increased participants' ability to narrate feelings and emotions about the troubling experiences encountered when seeking fertility treatment and adoption.

Maintaining a research log and using supervision when scheduled helped me to cope with unprocessed emotions and feelings. I found the research analysis and writing process both emotionally challenging and therapeutic. For example, through reflexive writing and analysis, I realised that the emotional demand I experienced was normal and that keeping an open mind facilitated my empowerment as a researcher. Initially, it was evident in my writing that my feelings directly affected my writing style. The ability to consciously negotiate and separate my practice and personal interests from the research role as I grew in confidence and was able to reflexively process feelings from the research interviews, allowed me to carefully and sensitively draw out important findings without being overly influenced by my personal or practitioner position.

Finlay (2002) argues that reflexivity is not about legitimised emoting but it develops insight about how the research space is managed and how this influences interpretation of data and research findings. The use of direct quotes to aid interpretation and meaning making was extremely powerful. This located the voice of the participants at the centre of their story/experience. Through self-reflective consciousness, I identified what my feelings were with regard to their experience, but also interpreted the meaning of the information and emotional reactions that had been reported (Finlay, 2002). I learnt that emotions cannot be shelved during research but can be used to enrich the analysis. And I came to appreciate that researching sensitive subjects is complex and unpredictable. I had to learn to manage my personal identity, professional identity and potential conflicts of interest between the researcher and professional role.

Researching PLWHIV constantly demanded sensitivity and active sensing of physical body responses as well as internal conversations. Although physical and verbal responses were evident as participants presented various emotions and feelings, these were absorbed within the interview room and transferred to my own 'container' of emotions. This emotional burden could not be avoided. I constantly questioned my responses, asking: is this the appropriate reaction? Is this the least destructive or the least harmful action? For me, being appropriate was about remaining neutral, fighting back tears and frustrations when listening to stories that were emotionally burdensome. I found that resisting the transference of the interviewee's feelings through reflexivity or counter-transference protected me as a researcher. I also learned that participants may empathise with researchers when they feel that their experience can be emotionally burdensome.

Strategies to Manage Reflexivity as a Researcher

- Clarify your own a priori conceptions.
- Allow data and the research process to trigger reflexive thoughts.
- Remain clear and focused on the research question when following participant stories and maintain an open attitude to participant responses.
- Have a clear researcher status and ability to adjust between conflicting roles to allow a transformation in self-identity as a researcher.
- Foster emotional resilience and find alternative confidential supervisory arrangements to address emotional disturbance during data collection.

Conclusion

This chapter explored processes used to engage in reflexive fieldwork when researching PLWHIV who experience HIV-induced infertility and seek adoption. I have described negotiating and renegotiating emotional and sensitive feelings and managing the boundary between researcher, practitioner relations. When tensions arise between the researcher or practitioner roles, personal or social relations can be managed through supervision, peer support and self sensitivity. Sensitive conscious engagement with data to account for a priori inferences with the interpretative process is important. In discussing these issues, I have emphasised that researching PLWHIV in a small research population may raise methodological and ethical challenges. It is also important to be open-minded, fluid and flexible about using alternative recruitment methods to manage ethical issues, boundaries and confidentiality.

References

Archer, M. S. (2010). *Conversations about reflexivity*. Oxon: Routledge.

Archer, M. S. (2012). *The reflexive imperative in late modernity*. New York: Cambridge University Press.

Binder, P., Holgersen, H., & Moltu, C. (2012). Staying close and reflexive: An explorative and reflexive approach to qualitative research on psychotherapy. *Nordic Psychology, 64*(2), 103–117.

Carroll, K. (2012). Infertile? The emotional labour of sensitive and feminist research methodologies. *Qualitative Research, 13*(5), 546–561.

Crossley, N. (2006). *Sociology and social change. Reflexive embodiment in contemporary society*. Berkshire: Open University Press.

Davies, C. A. (2008). *Reflexive ethnography. A guide to researching selves and others*. New York: Routledge.

Finlay, L. (2002). Negotiating the swamp: The opportunity and challenge of reflexivity in research practice. *Qualitative Research, 2*, 209–230.

Haggerty, K. D. (2004). Ethics creep: Governing social science research in the name of ethics. *Qualitative Sociology, 27*, 391.

Holmes, M. (2010). The emotionalization of reflexivity. *Sociology, 44*(1), 139–154.

Maccarini, A. M., & Prandini, R. (2010). Human reflexivity in social realism. In A. Archer (Ed.), *Conversations about reflexivity*. New York: Routledge.

Noble, K., & McIlveen, P. (2012). Being, knowing, and doing: A model for reflexivity in social constructionist practices. In P. McIlveen & D. E. Schultheiss (Eds.), *Social constructionism in vocational psychology and career development* (pp. 105–113). Rotterdam, Netherlands: Sense Publishers.

Ruch, G., & Julkunen, I. (2016). *Relationship-based research in social work: Understanding practice research*. London: Jessica Kingsley.

Sandelowski, M., & Barroso, J. (2002). Finding the findings in qualitative studies. *Journal of Nursing Scholarship, 34*(3), 213–220.

Savasi, V., Mandia, L., Laoreti, A., & Cetin, I. (2013). Reproductive assistance in HIV serodiscordant couples. *Human Reproduction Update, 19*(2), 136–150.

Skovdal, M., & Abebe, T. (2012). Reflexivity and dialogue: Methodological and socio-ethical dilemmas in research with HIV-affected children in East Africa. *Ethics, Policy and Environment, 15*(1), 77–96.

Smith, J. A. (2008). Reflecting on the development of interpretative phenomenological analysis and its contributions to qualitative research in psychology. *Qualitative Research in Psychology, 1*(1), 39–54.

Smith, J. A. (2012). Evaluating the contribution of interpretative phenomenological analysis. *Health Psychology Review, 5*(1), 9–27.

Smythe, E. A., Ironside, P. M., Sims, S. L., Swenson, M. M., & Spence, D. G. (2008). Doing Heideggerian hermeneutic research: A discussion paper. *International Journal of Nursing Studies, 45*(9), 1389–1397. https://doi.org/10.1016/j.ijnurstu.2007.09.005

Spence, D. G. (2016). Supervising for robust hermeneutic phenomenology: Reflexive engagement with horizons of understanding. *Qualitative Health Research*, 1–7. https://doi.org/10.1177/1049732316637824

Wiley, N. (2010). Inner speech and agency. In A. Archer (Ed.), *Conversation about reflexivity*. New York: Routledge.

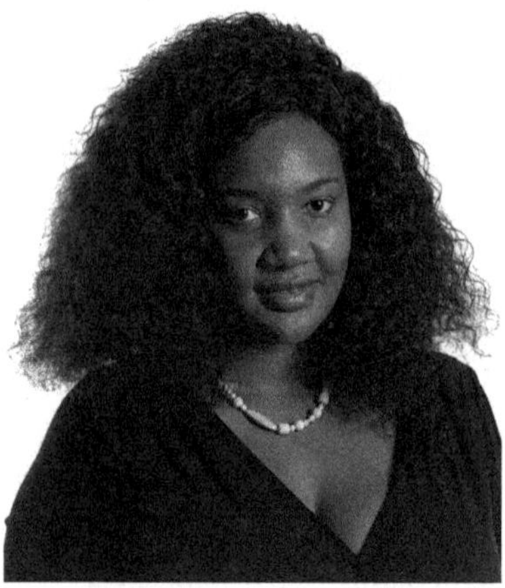

Tam Chipawe Cane is Senior Lecturer, Programme Leader for Social Work Programmes at the University of Greenwich, UK. She was awarded her clinical doctorate from the University of Surrey in 2015.

6

Fieldwork with Vulnerable Young People

Kit Tapson

Introduction

Although there are critics who consider reflection a contrived or self-affected indulgence (Finlay, 2002), for myself as a counsellor, reflexive practice facilitates reflection on my life and work experiences. Reflexivity is used to inform and enhance my practice and research as well as appraise the assumptions I hold (Boud & Fales, 1983; Boud, Keogh, & Walker, 1985; Mezirow, 1981; Jarvis, 1992). My work as both a counsellor and researcher requires reflexivity, enabling me to connect to my feelings and experiences in a way that enables me to *flex in action*. Flex in action is a fluid approach that allows me to respond to people and life situations in harmony with their circumstances, rather than in a rigid and unyielding manner. In this chapter, I discuss how I used reflexivity during my PhD and how I held the dual identities of researcher and counsellor. I begin with an introduction to my motivation to embark on the research and an outline of the study. I then discuss three incidents that challenged my reflexive awareness.

K. Tapson (✉)
Centre for Arts as Wellbeing, University of Winchester, Winchester, UK

H.T. Allan, A. Arber (eds.), *Emotions and reflexivity in Health and Social Care Field Research*, https://doi.org/10.1007/978-3-319-65503-1_6

Why Do the Study?

Before I began my research and whilst working as a counsellor in a practice located in a disadvantaged area, I was asked to undertake counselling sessions with young people who exhibited aggressive tendencies. On first meeting the young people, through their demeanour and body language, I felt a strong sense of threat. Undoubtedly, these feelings arose from previous reading of their character profiles. These profiles presented a summary of an assessment session which detailed the key reasons for why the young people sought counselling; these were mainly related to anger issues, and unpredictable tendencies to erupt. With understandable apprehension, not least for my own safety, I inevitably entered such sessions with preconceptions as to what could occur. However, once several sessions had elapsed, and we had begun to engage on a one-to-one basis, I noticed that close to the surface, and poorly constrained by their belligerent and hostile shell, a fragile and wretched vulnerability lurked close beneath the surface of many of the young people. This was highlighted when a young client, awarded an Anti-Social Behaviour Order for previous miscreant behaviour crumbled and cried when I showed compassion by communicating my desire to hear of his life experience; it appeared that he had never previously been asked to tell his life story. This event triggered me to reflect on both the nature of the client/counsellor relationship in such circumstances and also the response of counsellors to this client group. It was the generation of this intense interest, along with a continuing concern for the young people that I counselled, that called out to me as a practitioner and actually represented the first step towards becoming a researcher. The research problem then became: how do counsellors connect with the core of this injured group in a way that enables change?

In my research I sought to authentically represent the young people's perspectives as well as the counsellor's perspective in the hope that what inhibits and facilitates the therapeutic relationship with young people who bully would extend understanding for practice. The research was conducted using interpretative phenomenological analysis (IPA), which assumes a critical realist position, meaning there are stable and enduring features of reality that exist independently of human conceptualisation

(Smith, 2004). However, the meaning of the reality varies according to how individuals experience it (Ackroyd, 2004), since each brings varying evaluative and self-reflective capacities. For the researcher, temporarily inhabiting and understanding participants' meanings requires intersubjectivity, or the ability to share more than one conscious mind. I chose a methodological approach based on critical realism because of my counselling experiences with young people who bullied. In my counselling work, I was aware of a gap between my worldview and that of young people themselves, in other words multiple world views. The gap between my world view and the young people was obvious in counselling sessions, where young people described their lived experiences using dark and foreboding language, such as 'empty, depressed and pointless', creating a picture of a black and dispirited existence.

A central assumption of IPA is that the researcher brings their own unbracketed experiences to their work (Giorgi, 2008), helping contextualise phenomena in both a personal and social setting (Ashworth, 2006; King et al., 2008). For example, having been bullied during childhood for my prodigious outcrop of freckles, I was conscious that any anger lingering from my own lived experience may manifest as resentment towards the young people who bully. In fact, it was not until the data gathering period that my resentment took shape, a response triggered by a seemingly dismissive comment by Andy about people deserving to be bullied. This affronted my historical, but apparently unresolved, victim status. This realisation triggered two lines of thought. Firstly, it made me question the authenticity of my motivation to study young people who bully. Secondly, it emphasised the importance of mandatory counselling for all trainee counsellors such that internalised assumptions can be explored in a safe environment. Resolving the dilemma was not easy as it had taken form in a dynamic and unforgiving setting. The only solution was to view the event as an opportunity for advanced reflection and personal growth, but I remain unsure as to how successful or sustainable these strategies proved since objectivity may have been hindered by the context. With the researcher inextricably linked to the phenomenon under study in this way, my position and assumptions inevitably influenced data collection and interpretation.

Understandably then, Smith and Pietkiewicz (2008) comment that whilst importing the researcher's un-bracketed assumptions which may enrich the gathering and interpretation of data, it creates a locus demanding advanced self-awareness; particularly with disadvantaged groups, to avoid disempowerment. There was a strong awareness of disempowerment in my practice as a counsellor and of the power relations between researcher and researched in work with young people from disadvantageous backgrounds which formed an important element of the research process. My awareness and the empathy I shared with the young people and counsellors meant there was some integration here of Finlay's 4th method of reflexivity: social critique. This of course was not openly spoken about but occurred at the unconscious level.

So whilst IPA entrusts the researcher to use their assumptions to enlighten understanding of the participants' perceptions of phenomena, negative preconceptions from my own experiences of being bullied may easily, unconsciously, have predisposed me to interpret the young people's narrative with prejudice. This, I argue, placed me in a powerful position, as analysis of the participant's narrative rested with my experiences, and was therefore precarious. As Hunt (1989, p. 218) observes: "[…] who am I, simply by dint of my training, to be so sure when interpreting another's world? I am uncomfortable about the power I assume when explaining others' motives". Later in the chapter I discuss occasions where my assumptions became entangled in the participant/researcher relationship.

I recruited young people aged 11–18 years, who were identified as having a tendency to bully and who had received no less than three one-to-one counselling sessions with a professional counsellor. After some discussion with various agencies, access to participants was ultimately negotiated through two part-charitable and part-council run projects, both of which offered learning support and counselling to young people exhibiting aggression and behavioural problems. I managed to consent four young people (Jason, Andy, Courtney and Lucy) and their two counsellors to the study.

The Study

The research design was qualitative, starting with an eighteen-month period of informal observation where for two hours each week, I joined the young people in their classroom setting at one of the centres. Whilst the observation periods were not used as data, and consent was not required, I recorded my thoughts and feelings in a reflective journal, which I later used as a tool to deepen the analysis. An overriding impression from this journal in the subsequent analysis was of the intense resistance the young people brought to all activities and relationships, opposing their teachers, confronting their peers and even battling their own emotions. An example is when the young people were receiving sex education:

> The teacher hands out a selection of condoms to the young people with the intention of demonstrating how these should be worn. But a splinter group sitting on the settees in the recreation area, get out their lighters, make a pile from the condoms, and set fire to them causing a cloud of acrid smoke that fills the classroom. After extinguishers have been used to subdue the fire, the teacher voices her dispiritedness that all her careful lesson preparation has been reduced to nothing. (Reflective Journal)

I felt fearful of the young people's determined obstructiveness, not only because of the intense anger that seemed to fuel it, but also because of the inevitable struggle to gather data that their antagonism portended. Such challenge was unfortunately realised in the data collection phase when in focus groups, the determined anger of two of the participants caused them to fiercely defend against questions as to their counselling experiences. They perceived my questions as intrusive; this resistant attitude on several occasions caused the focus groups to grind to a halt. This left us all sitting in prolonged silence and I was reluctant to interrupt in case any sense of discomfort was mine alone. I interpreted these resistances as data using psychodynamic theory (see Jacobs, 1999; Walkerdine, Lucey, & Melody, 2001). The observations provided a glimpse of how the young people interacted in their familiar environment, their attitude to education, social skills and behaviour, but most importantly, it provided the opportunity for building trust with them. I reflected that for the counsellors whose work centred on young people who bully, building trust was not an easy undertaking as the damage the young people had incurred left them wounded such that any approach they perceived as a threat would cause them to back away. I understood that a safer tactic for the young people was to leave them to come to me, to signal their own readiness to engage and provide an opening for me to bond in their own territory and time.

Following the period of informal observation, I conducted two focus groups with four young people and two focus groups with the counsellors. In addition, I conducted two semi-structured individual interviews with each counsellor, where their separation from each other facilitated very different accounts from those at the focus groups. For example, whilst together, the counsellors were insistent that they remained calm in the face of their continual contact with aggressive clients. In individual interviews, one counsellor disclosed the emotional drain of her work. These two forms of interview offered different positions for viewing the world, and I go on to discuss this later in the chapter.

Reliability was a consideration in my study, especially as IPA does not seek consistency or measurability. Moreover, validity represents how well research reflects the reality it claims to represent, and yet, the critical realist stance of IPA disputes the notion of one unequivocal reality, proposing instead that interpretation of reality is dependent upon the lived experiences of the perceiver. Smith (2011) proposes that methodological rigour is achieved through credibility and trustworthiness, a process dependent upon plausible and persuasive evidence to support interpretation of the data. For me, reflexivity involves using my integrity to negotiate meanings, to analyse the objective, subjective and intersubjective elements of the narrative I share with the participants; to realise a responsible representation of our words and emotions. As such, I kept both a reflective and research journal. The reflective journal was used to record my thoughts and feelings about the research process whereas the research journal was used to document practical elements of the study, details about settings, location and contacts. Material from both sources was combined to provide an accurate overview of the study. Additionally, I inserted my thoughts within the transcripts when analysing the data, cross-referencing entries from the reflective journal and the transcripts to aid interpretation. These sources were supplemented by reference to fieldnotes where the research data had been recorded. During analysis when I thought I had recalled events with accuracy, I realised I had sometimes overlooked details of the setting or the intensity of my feelings from observing certain incidents. Constant comparison between the two journals and the fieldnotes countered potential lapses in memory. As recommended by Smith (2003), interpretation of the data was further verified by my supervisors through an 'independent audit' (p. 234). During these sessions my two supervisors and I would carefully analyse and pull apart sections of the data and my journals, using our expertise including our clinical experience, mental health experience and research experience.

In the next section I discuss a fight observed between two of the young people during the initial observation period. I reflect upon the impact of the event upon my dual identity as a researcher and counsellor and the reflexive awareness used to make sense of the incidence, which shook and challenged my beliefs.

Responding to Aggression in the Field

During my first morning of observation at Centre A I noticed mounting tension in the bodies of two boys, Andy and Jason. Both came from deprived backgrounds and had been victims to dysfunctional parenting from an early age. Apart from experiencing Attention Deficit Hyperactivity Disorder (ADHD)[1] they were defensive and aggressive in their relationships with others, and their disclosures during observation revealed they had a damaged self-worth. On this occasion, Andy had squared his shoulders, was clenching and unclenching his fists, whilst Jason leant slightly backward in his chair. Although the staff at Centre A appeared oblivious to this bodily expression, as a counsellor I am highly attuned to non-verbal language. As a newcomer, and non-participant observer, I felt powerless to contravene the boundaries of my research identity. Suddenly, the tables separated, Andy fell upon Jason, beating him savagely, knocking out two teeth and breaking Jason's nose. Staff attempted to diffuse the boys' fury using recognised anger management techniques without success; the boys, particularly Andy, attempted to resume the fight at every opportunity for a while. On the drive home, I realised I was shaking both as a release of the fear I had internalised and also from indignation at Andy's behaviour. I also recognised that the source of this indignation may have lodged with a lingering bias from my experience as a victim of bullying; I realised I had unwittingly labelled Andy as persecutor. Being a novice researcher, it did not cross my mind to seek support following this event. It was not until I received academic supervision at the university that I retold the practical details of what had occurred. Despite realising that I had embodied stress, I did not disclose this to my supervisors, assuming that emotional anxiety was an expected bi-product of researching vulnerable groups.

Faced with Andy's savagery, it was challenging for me to justify his behaviour. I had witnessed him beating another person, as if possessed by a ferocious and mindless aggression. When recording the fight in my journal later that day, I was shocked and disappointed to realise that from reading back over my words, I had abandoned the more empathic rationale of my counsellor identity (which would have meant conceptualising his damaged development). Instead I was thinking of Andy as a thug. This realisation made me question the foundations of my being as a counsellor, and also my un-bracketed assumptions, since how I had co-constructed my participant's phenomenon was imbued with personal prejudices. Had I broached these uncertainties with my supervisors, they would undoubtedly have been attentive. I think I was inhibited from sharing these doubts by my British 'stiff upper lip', and believing I had to internalise my worries and deal with them alone. I was not receiving supervision as a counsellor at this time.

To ground this experience, I consulted instead what is known in the world of counselling as the 'internal supervisor', a "friendly super-ego that can be referred to at times when formal supervision is unavailable" (Rickard, 2012), to offer an inner locus of evaluation (Rogers, 1951). I recalled what staff at Centre A had told me of Andy's childhood, how he had been provoked and beaten by his parents, realising upon reflection that he was possessed, not by a pointless aggression, but overwhelmed by an impotent anger. I realised that the rules which formed the scaffold of Andy's feelings were far removed from my own. Conceiving of Andy as a thug had been a statement of my fear, affording me a temporary but blind alignment with the safety of shared societal values; a collective response so similar to that of young people who bully when under threat. I felt forced to reflect on uncomfortable personal insights, whilst unveiling a complex ideological agenda hidden within the text. Bruner (1986, p. 150) argues that at these times, the researcher "appears not as an individual creative scholar, a knowing subject who discovers, but more as a material body through whom a narrative structure unfolds". Following this event, I wondered how, or even if, the counsellors manage to maintain calm when faced with angry young people on a daily basis.

Maintaining Calm

Shocked at the power of my personal prejudices to temporarily blind me to compassion and empathy, and scared at my own reactions to the violence I had observed both as a counsellor and a researcher, I was surprised by a conversation with counsellors A and B in the focus groups. I asked the counsellors how, faced with young people who bully on a daily basis, they managed their own emotions. They both maintained they felt a consistent calm that surprised me.

> Researcher: [...] you frequently alluded to remaining calm as an essential component of your counselling, with relation to stabilising your clients. But what effect, if any, does remaining calm have upon your clients?
>
> Counsellor A: What effect does it have upon my clients? I think being calm allows me to calmly assess the client, assess the situation, think about what they're saying. And, if I wasn't calm, I wouldn't be able to process that much information all at the same time.
>
> Researcher: I mean, I guess the angle that I'm coming from is…um…do you need to stay calm to provide yourself with some sort of framework so that you don't get overwhelmed with the work?
>
> Counsellor A: No. I don't ever feel overwhelmed in the room. I might do afterwards sometimes, but not in the room. Well, maybe then, the answer is yes, because that's why I don't get overwhelmed in the room, because I…I am able to stay calm in the room. And it's almost like a natural, instinctive thing that happens in the room. Um…not to say that I don't get emotional in the room. I do, often, but I'm still emotionally calm.

Seemingly, Counsellors A and B possessed emotional management skills far in advance of my own. In hindsight, I realised that I was motivated to seek their opinions about emotions to validate my own abilities as I had unconsciously hoped that they too would 'confess' to struggling when faced with aggressive clients. In addition, I hoped that hearing of Counsellor A and B's experiences of maintaining calm may help me come to terms with the episode with Andy, which had certainly threatened my sense of competence as a counsellor. Attempting to make sense of these unanticipated data, I came across Hochschild's work. Hochschild (1983) sees the self as moderated by social influence according to 'feeling rules' (Hochschild, 1998, p. 242) which shape emotions and how these are expressed. Therefore, emotional management is influenced according to the kind of emotion experienced and how that experience is conceptualised according to the values and norms concerning feeling. In other words, how feelings are managed can both affect and effect emotion.

> Within organisational contexts, the appropriation of emotions undergoes further management known as emotional labour, since how feelings are experienced and expressed must be in keeping with the values of the organisation, but also in a way that "produces a proper state of mind in others" (Hochschild, 1983, p. 7). This is achieved by suppressing unpalatable feelings (like anger) to replace them with more acceptable feelings (like sympathy). In relation to Counsellor A and B's calm countenance, Hochschild's (1983, 1998) theory suggested their emotional management was the unconscious suppression of negative feelings towards their clients, replaced with a calm identity more in-keeping with societal expectations about counsellors. In the face of my professional disquiet when faced with aggressive clients, compared to the counsellor's claims of calm, I thought emotional management was something I did not own.

In contrast to Hochschild, Freud ([2001] 1923) considered repressed emotions as too volatile and unpredictable to be successfully suppressed, suggesting instead that they would emerge without mediation by either social factors or their owner. This interpretation seemed to make more sense when reading my data. For instance, when describing how she challenged angry clients who bully in what she identified as a "[…] calm way […]" Counsellor B's example of interacting with her aggressive clients suggested sentiments at variance with her avowal of calm:

> Counsellor B: 'You're not bullying me! I'm not impressed. Let's just calm down and we'll start this one again'. And sometimes that's necessary to just sort of lower the temperature and say….you know, 'sit down! I can't talk to you while you're pacing the room. Sit down. If I can't hear you, why are you shouting at me?' (Transcript focus group 2. Counsellors B)

Counsellor B appeared unaware of the anger in her voice, and I sensed a volatile emotion had unpredictably been vocalised without censorship. Counsellor B was not alone, for when talking about presenting a client to her supervisor, Counsellor A seemed likewise to have repressed some anger:

> Counsellor A: I was literally, stood up in the room, walking round the room, doing the little voice (said in a whisper), getting louder and louder and louder (her volume increases) until I was shouting…
>
> Researcher: How did you feel after you had re-enacted your client in that way?
>
> Counsellor A: I could let go then. Yeah. Let go of that... Yeah. (Transcript. Focus group 4. Counsellors A and B)

Since I had recorded in my reflective journal how Counsellor A's shoulders sagged whilst speaking, the 'letting go' to which she referred suggested to me relief from holding an unwieldy package. It was difficult not to interpret this narrative as implying that the weight of her client's anger had indeed been repressed by Counsellor A but had leaked through a fissure during her re-enactment at supervision. Whilst supervision provides a safe forum for counsellors to review their work in order to learn from experience (Carroll, 2007), it is not always considered a reliable setting for the expression or exploration of unconscious forces. According to Erskine, Moursund, and Trautmann (1999), supervisors have their own blind spots which can leave them oblivious to the repressed emotions of their supervisees in clinical supervision and it is interesting to note that following her emotional outburst, Counsellor A described how her supervisor 'just sat there' (Transcript. Focus group 3. Counsellors A and B) which I interpreted as the supervisor not recognising the transference and counter-transference.

Considering the counsellors in light of emotional management did not come without concern though, as I was reluctant to simply import a theory into the research encounter without question, particularly one that challenged the roots of their therapeutic work. To explain what is meant by this latter point, I can only refer to the work of Carl Rogers whose insightful writing and life-long dedication to the therapeutic relationship have brought wisdom to bear on the topic. Rogers (1992) was of the opinion that for the client to effect change, six conditions should exist, number five being that "The therapist experiences an empathic understanding of the client's internal frame of reference and endeavours to communicate this experience to the client" (p. 828). Consequently, I questioned how this basic and essential connection could be made if Counsellors A and B were shielded from the rawness of their client's aggression by their reported cloak of calm.

In relation to my dual identity as researcher/counsellor, the issues raised by this example of emotional management are important. A founding principle of counselling, and a recognised ethical guideline, is to do the client no harm. And yet I reasoned that although Counsellor A and B's insistence on calm was an understandable distancing tactic that may offer self-protection from exposure to their aggressive clients, it may also inhibit the client from authentic expression. According to Winnicott (1994) muffling or repressing the genuine emotions of clients who are angry or who bully could even constrain their development. Winnicott proposed that, to analyse 'antisocials', the analyst must "sort out and study his objective reactions to the patient" (p. 351). This was important as the patient could only appreciate in the analyst what he (the analyst) was capable of feeling (Winnicott, 1994). So, for example, with patients experiencing love/hate states, should the analyst show only love or hate, they would be capable of 'killing the patient' (Winnicott, 1994, p. 351). Hence, Winnicott warned that the analyst must not deny that hate existed within them but rather, that hate, justified in the present context, must be identified and kept available for eventual interpretation. As a researcher it was not my responsibility to take action in this matter but as a caring and morally responsible counsellor, I felt a professional commitment to my practitioner identity and found myself suspended between these two roles in an 'I don't know' position. The impact of this dilemma should not be underestimated and it is only in retrospect that I realised the severity of the stress I experienced, as I oscilated between the duties to uphold my practice values compared to the more objectified profile as researcher. This experience represented a quandary for, when attempting to withhold myself as counsellor and analyse the data as purely a researcher, I felt compromised and unable to engage with the data. The double hermeneutic in IPA describes the use of self as an instrument in both the telling of the participant's story and interpretation of the emergent themes (Smith, 2004). But Giorgi (1994) questions the extent to which the researcher is present in this undertaking, recommending that some objectivity is needed to make sense of subjectivity.

As researcher/counsellor I was constantly aware of my responsibilities in both positions. For example, I was continually disturbed by the vulnerability of the young participants and stirred to respond as a counsellor. Dickson-Swift, James, Kippen, and Liamputtong (2006) observe that a fundamental challenge in this dual role position is in differentiating between research and therapy; since as qualitative researchers, we have to be ready to face human feelings (Ely, Anzul, Friedman, Garner, & Steinmetz, 1991). However, responding with empathy and caring threatened to blur the boundaries between the participants and myself. Managing the emotions of the young people sometimes came at a personal cost since I was alert to the damage they had incurred in their lives and felt a huge responsibility to safeguard their fragility and facilitate the trust between us that would enable them to share their stories. But in listening to their powerful accounts, I absorbed their voices, replaying sentences in my mind throughout the day, hearing their weighty sadness. This emotional experience was like wearing a mantle throughout data gathering; a metaphorical *overcoat* that I later realised hid my feelings. Once again, I did not reveal these emotions to my supervisors as I understood supervision to be more an academic support than an emotional one. An additional buffer was that, like Counsellors A and B, in the quest for objectivity, I sometimes abandoned my counsellor identity, deferring instead to theory and protocol as protective armour from subjectivity; an example of how emotional management influenced the enactment of my dual identities after all.

Being a counsellor/researcher was therefore both an advantage and a disadvantage as although there were undoubtedly instances when our understanding converged, there were equally times of divergence. By questioning the counsellors' calm tactics I had imported a practitioner agenda that made comparison with my own counselling experiences, and one which threatened to prioritise my practice above my research identity. In terms of their therapeutic work, I had anticipated that for the counsellors, as for myself, that the aggressive attitude of the young people who bullied would occasionally permeate their professional persona, ruffling, or even scaring them. Although using IPA, the self-in relation-to-others becomes both the aim and object of focus, I realised I had to avoid assuming a mutual understanding of our work, since our oppositional interpretation of the therapeutic relationship had highlighted that it was this very awareness that enabled identification of our differences. Such advanced mindfulness of the practitioner/researcher boundaries demands considerable emotional energy, linking directly to the beginning of this paragraph and the fight between Jason and Andy, where the awareness needed to safeguard my researcher identity overwhelmed my instincts to act as a counsellor. It is also possible that adopting the researcher identity on this occasion felt like the safer option.

Resistance and a Fragile Sense of Self

Confused as to the dual but conflicting roles of being a counsellor and researcher, I sought guidance as to the characteristics defining these two professions from accessing their regulatory frameworks online. Rather than providing clarity however, this exercise further muddied the waters since both professions appeared regulated by similar ethical principles; fundamentally, an overwhelming commitment to participant beneficence, safeguarding confidentiality and respecting anonymity (BACP, 2015; ESRC, 2016). It was these similarities that triggered particular anxiety with Andy during the course of data gathering.

Coming from a troubled home, Andy had crafted an exterior that contradicted the mess in his life forming an essential fortress to protect him from harm. Leaning back in his chair, Andy exhibited little fallibility, enacting a disengaged character, appearing to be unruffled by life. The phrase 'too cool for school' appeared to be his mantra. However, I noticed that Andy seldom engaged eye contact and constantly fidgeted with his hands. Although his frequent response to discussion 'I dunno' implied a need for distance, he unwittingly *leaked*[2] a desire to be liked. For example, when discussing his counselling during a focus group, Andy commented:

> Andy: Well, it's a waste of time isn't it? : I just sit there. I bin a couple of times. I just sit there and say like stupid things like to make them happy. Then they say I'm good. (Transcript. Focus group 1. Young people)

A phenomenological reading of Andy's experience of counselling suggested he was not committed to the process, he was there for the counsellor's benefit. He seemed to hint at his self-worth. However, conflict appeared in this sentence as it had in previous disclosures, as it seemed the personal gain he acknowledged came not from subjective change, but from the accolade afforded him by his counsellors identifying him as good.

At his disclosure, I felt palpable sadness for Andy, a sense of isolation at the dereliction of his sense of self and the erection of his nonchalance, a fragile shell encasing his need to be liked. From my observations and his words I felt he appeared to live in parallel worlds; one in which he existed for the sole purpose of the feelings and needs of others. And the other where he experienced profound loneliness and emptiness. Had he visited me as a client, I would have taken time to develop a safe and trusting relationship that paid tribute to the private and personal part of him he was revealing in the focus groups. Yet as researcher, I was aware not only of the problematic boundary issues of tipping into a therapeutic relationship with Andy, but also the limited attention span of the young people, whose ADHD made prolonged concentration challenging for them. As such, it was necessary to temporarily set aside my counsellor identity and push through the boundaries in a way that at times felt insensitive and rough. For example, during one focus group, Andy commented that he would tell his counsellor nothing, "not even if [he] cut [his] finger" (Transcript 1. Focus group 1). Despite the fact that Andy had been abused and emotionally neglected during his development, his decision to withhold a 'cut finger' from his counsellor evoked a powerful narrative of his fragility as an injured child. I felt a physical ache at Andy's vulnerable self-worth and his need for affirmation. Trawling through my own lived experience to locate the source of these feelings, I was reminded of my first days at school, my home sickness and missing my Mother. It was only in this way that I could fully empathise with how, for Andy, his specific understanding of reality had found form and how the connections between subject and object had, for him, taken shape. I later realised that I had unknowingly embraced the essence of IPA, rooted as it is in critical realism. I was able to briefly enter the social and emotional world of the participants; an intersubjective experience that provided a fleeting glimpse of his reality. With no time to explore this sorrowful disclosure, Andy's sensitive emotions were lost in the on-going group narrative. I reflected how this dilemma may have been resolved had I not been a counsellor, and yet it was precisely the qualities of heightened awareness, empathy and unconditional positive regard which Rogers (1992) considers to define the therapist, that had alerted me to Andy's lived experiences in the first place. The conflict of my dual identity was further tested when writing the events of the day in my reflective journal, I was shocked at my evaluation of Andy's words as meaty data that would benefit my PhD. I would not have expressed that attitude whilst working as a counsellor. I felt shamed by this revelation: by temporarily misplacing the beneficence of the client or participant, I had abandoned the core of both counselling and research. The incident was a learning point since I realised that authenticity in relationship with another is an on-going negotiation of truth and congruence in both research and counselling.

Whilst planning my PhD, I gave considerable thought to the ethical safety and welfare of the participants, and little to my own, possibly, underestimating how impactful the young peoples' distress would be. Apart from the support from my academic supervisors, I sought no other. To cope with the emotional risks, some authors have suggested that researchers should be encouraged to seek supervision outside of the university setting (See for example, Etherington, 1996; Hubbard, Backett-Milburn, & Kemmer, 2001). Etherington (1996) points out that "as counsellors, we take this for granted; as researchers it is equally important" (p. 346). In addition, the non-directive nature of qualitative research, such as this study means that I entered the field with little control over the participants' narratives, providing instead a fluid space for them to tell their stories, but sometimes journeying to places I was not prepared for. In this respect, the intensity of the young peoples' anger was the most threatening emotion I experienced. Dickson-Swift, James, Kippen, and Liamputtong (2007) considers supervision as important in supporting researchers to manage the challenges of sensitive studies and that to enhance the researcher's abilities and protect their well-being, sessions could be used to debrief, mentor and develop the skills of researchers. Whilst I was fortunate in having attentive supervisors, I nonetheless carried the young people's stories around with me and appreciate how this may have undermined my emotional well-being (Warr, 2004).

Strategies for Reflexivity in the Field

From the events reflected upon in the current chapter, I can only conclude that being a counsellor and researcher has been both advantageous and problematic. Although my therapeutic training may well have facilitated a safe space in which the participants felt better able to disclose, the conflict has been in listening to their sad tales without reaching out to explore the young peoples' troubles and offer compassion. I would suggest the following strategies to other researchers when planning and conducting research:

- Find support during fieldwork involving intense suffering and social injustice.
- Fostering relationships with fellow students can be a source of comfort.
- Academic supervisors should be attentive to the well-being of vulnerable researchers.
- Create space for recovery: leave time between emotionally charged interviews and focus groups.
- Awareness of the difficulties posed by having a dual identity could be usefully explored during the training of professional researchers.
- Considerable thought needs to be given to continuing clinical supervision.

Conclusions

For me, an enduring question is how I can trust my intuitive self to know if my interpretation of others' experiences is authentic. Atkins and Murphy (1993), consider reflection is triggered by discomfort or curiosity. In the case of Andy, it was my uneasiness at affording him a convenient social label that initiated critical analysis of my thoughts and feelings. This research experience taught me that reflexivity often starts by attending to our most basic feelings. Had I approached data gathering by bracketing these feelings, as prescribed by Husserl (1983), I may have lacked awareness of the pre-existing beliefs which were ultimately to benefit me, as they were re-evaluated in the light of emerging data and the phenomenon under investigation. Reflexivity opened a window onto my knowledge and personal assumptions in a way that nurtured empathy. Reflexivity facilitated a new perspective as to the subjective and objective enmeshment of reality for young people who bully, nurturing new learning but also highlighting that personal reflection is limited by one's own understanding and experiences. It is not sufficient simply to report and describe data, but to weave both a portrait and a landscape of our participants and ourselves that enhances transparency, trustworthiness, and our own accountability. The supervisor's role is vital, since encouraging reflexivity, accountability and responsibility helps to build knowledge about the emotional risks experienced by the researcher when undertaking sensitive research.

Notes

1. In people with ADHD sustained focus represents a significant challenge.
2. Leaking an emotion unconsciously.

References

Ackroyd, S. (2004). Methodology for management and organisation studies: Some implications of critical realism. In S. Fleetwood & S. Ackroyd (Eds.), *Critical realist applications in organisation and management studies* (pp. 137–163). London and New York: Routledge.

Ashworth, P. D. (2006). Seeing oneself as a carer in the activity of caring. Attending to the lifeworld of the person with Alzheimer's disease. *International Journal of Qualitative Studies in Health and Well-being, 1*(4), 212–225.

Atkins, T. W., & Murphy, K. (1993). Reflection: A review of the literature. *Journal of Advanced Nursing, 18*, 1188–1192.

Boud, D., & Fales, A. (1983). Reflective learning: Key to learning from experience. *Journal of Humanistic Psychology, 23*(2), 99–117.

Boud, D., Keogh, R., & Walker, D. (1985). Promoting reflection in learning: A model. In D. Boud, R. Keogh, & D. Walker (Eds.), *Reflection: Turning experience into learning* (pp. 18–40). London: Kogan Page.

British Association for Counselling and Psychotherapy (BACP). (2015). *Ethical framework for good practice in counselling and psychotherapy.* Retrieved from the British Association for Counselling and Psychotherapy website: http://www.bacp.co.uk/events/learning_programmes/ethical_framework/documents/ethical_framework_mono.pdf

Bruner, E. M. (1986). Ethnography as narrative. In V. Turner & E. Bruner (Eds.), *The anthropology of experience* (pp. 3–385). Chicago: University of Illinois Press.

Carroll, M. (2007). One more time: What is supervision? *Psychotherapy in Australia, 13*(3), 34–40.

Dickson-Swift, V., James, E., Kippen, S., & Liamputtong, P. (2006). Blurring boundaries in qualitative health research on sensitive topics. *Qualitative Health Research, 16*, 853–871.

Dickson-Swift, V., James, E., Kippen, S., & Liamputtong, P. (2007). Doing sensitive research: What challenges do qualitative researchers face? *Qualitative Research, 7*(3), 327–353.

Economic and Social Research Council. (2016). *Policies and standards.* Retrieved from the Economic and Social Research Council website: http://www.esrc.ac.uk/about-us/policies-and-standards/

Ely, M., Anzul, M., Friedman, T., Garner, D., & Steinmetz, A. (1991). *Doing qualitative research: Circles within circles.* London: Falmer Press.

Erskine, R. G., Moursund, J. P., & Trautmann, R. L. (1999). *Beyond empathy. A therapy of contact-in-relationship*. Philadelphia: Brunner/Mazel.

Etherington, K. (1996). The counsellor as researcher: Boundary issues and critical dilemmas. *British Journal of Guidance & Counselling, 24*(3), 339–346.

Finlay, L. (2002). Negotiating the swamp: The opportunity and challenge of reflexivity in research practice. *Qualitative Research, 2*(2), 209–230.

Freud, S. ([2001] 1923). The ego and the id. In S. L. Cavanagh, A. Failler & R. Alpha, J. Hurst (Eds.), *Skin, culture and psychoanalysis* (pp 106-121). London: Palgrave Macmillan.

Giorgi, A. (1994). A phenomenological perspective on certain qualitative research methods. *Journal of Phenomenological Psychology, 25*, 190–220.

Giorgi, A. (2008). Difficulties encountered in the application of the phenomenological method in the social sciences. *The Indo-Pacific of Phenomenology, 8*(1), 1–9.

Hochschild, A. R. (1983). *The managed heart.* Berkeley: University of California Press.

Hochschild, A. R. (1998). The sociology of emotion as a way of seeing. In G. Bendelow & S. J. Williams (Eds.), *Emotions in social life: Critical themes and contemporary issues.* London: Routledge.

Hubbard, G., Backett-Milburn, K., & Kemmer, D. (2001). Working with emotions: Issues for the researcher in fieldwork and teamwork. *International Journal of Social Research Methodology, 4*(2), 119–137.
Hunt, J. C. (1989). *Psychoanalytic aspects of fieldwork. Qualitative research methods 18*. Newbury Park, CA: Sage.
Husserl, E. (1983). *Ideas pertaining to a pure phenomenology and to a phenomenological philosophy*. The Hague: Martinus Nijhoff Publishers.
Jacobs, M. (1999). *Psychodynamic counselling in action* (3rd ed.). London: Sage.
Jarvis, P. (1992). Reflective practice and nursing. *Nurse Education Today, 12*(3), 174–181.
King, N., Finlay, L., Ashworth, P., Smith, J. A., Langdridge, D., & Butt, T. (2008). Can't really trust that, so what can I trust?' A polyvocal, qualitative analysis of the psychology of mistrust. *Qualitative Research in Psychology, 5*(2), 80–102.
Mezirow, J. (1981). A critical theory of adult learning and education. *Adult Education, 32*(1), 3–24.
Rickard, A. (2012). The internal supervisor. *Therapy Today, 22*(1), 26.
Rogers, C. R. (1951). *Client centred therapy: Its current practice. Implications and theory*. London: Constable and Company.
Rogers, C. R. (1992). The necessary and sufficient conditions of therapeutic personality change. *Journal of Consulting and Clinical Psychology, 60*(6), 827–832.
Smith, J. A. (2003). Validity and qualitative psychology. In J. A. Smith (Ed.), *Qualitative psychology. A practical guide to research methods* (pp. 232–235). London: Sage.
Smith, J. A. (2004). Reflecting on the development of interpretative phenomenological analysis and its contribution to qualitative research in psychology. *Qualitative Research in Psychology, 1*(1), 39–54.
Smith, J. A. (2011). Evaluating the contribution of interpretative phenomenological analysis. *Health Psychology Review, 5*(1), 9–27.
Smith, J. A., & Pietkiewicz, I. (2008). A practical guide to using interpretative phenomenological analysis in qualitative research psychology. *Psychological Journal, 18*(2), 361–369.
Walkerdine, V., Lucey, H., & Melody, J. (2001). *Growing up girl: Psychosocial explorations of gender and class*. Basingstoke: Palgrave.
Warr, D. (2004). Stories in the flesh and voices in the head: Reflections on the context and impact of research with disadvantaged populations. *Qualitative Health Research, 14*, 578–587.
Winnicott, D. W. (1994). Hate in the countertransference. *Journal of Psychotherapy Practice and Research, 3*(4), 350–356.

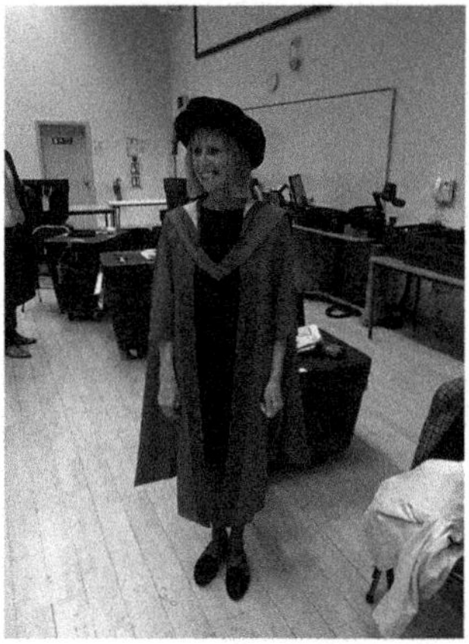

Kit Tapson is a research fellow at the Centre for Arts and Wellbeing, University of Winchester, UK. She was awarded her clinical doctorate from the University of Surrey in 2015.

7

Fieldwork in Other Cultures

Nicola Ayers

Introduction

What is it like to be a researcher in a different culture when everything seems unfamiliar? The aim of this chapter is to explore the emotional experiences and challenges faced whilst conducting fieldwork in Addis Ababa, Ethiopia. This chapter will focus on the complexities I faced when beginning my research and the stumbling blocks whilst conducting an ethnography overseas. I describe the practical steps I took to be reflexive, for example when taking on the roles of insider and outsider. The importance of regular supervision, where supervisors monitor the quality of the fieldwork data and raise awareness of the pull to 'going native', is explored. My experiences of many stumbling blocks were challenging, and as a result, I needed to develop skills in emotion work, emotional awareness and reflexivity to both support the research process and provide methodologically rich data.

N. Ayers (✉)
Federal Ministry of Health, Addis Ababa, Ethiopia

H.T. Allan, A. Arber (eds.), *Emotions and reflexivity in Health and Social Care Field Research*, https://doi.org/10.1007/978-3-319-65503-1_7

Background to the Study

The process of death and dying is unique from culture to culture. How people deal with pain, the rituals surrounding the dying process and what is perceived as a good death are all jointly constructed meanings made by a society through cultural practices (Seale, 1998). Death and dying can be seen as an interaction between the particular social structures of society, relationships and the body. For example, a society may be, traditional or modern, collective or individualistic, relationships may include those between family, friends, community and medical staff (Walter, 1994). The process of dying, as the body deteriorates, provokes a reaction in a society that is 'culturally shaped' (Seale, 1998, p. 49). My Ph.D. explored cultural practices around dying within the emerging palliative care service in Addis Ababa.

As the aim of the study was to research cultural beliefs, I thought a qualitative stance was the most appropriate approach; little was known about the emerging palliative care movement in Addis Ababa, and a focus on this development offered an interesting topic for my research. The aim of the study was to explore the care of the dying and to investigate the experiences of patients, carers and staff within their cultural context. I considered that ethnography was a methodological fit, as the premise of this study is linked to the cultural implications care of the dying in this setting. Ethnography has been portrayed as 'the art and science of describing a group or culture' (Fetterman, 2009, p. 1). Ethnography has historically been used to research the unfamiliar, but it is also now used to examine familiar surroundings.

As ethnography has developed it has taken on various forms. For the purpose of this study a 'focused ethnography' was the most appropriate because as Knoblauch (2005, p. 11) suggests, focused ethnographies study the 'situative performance of social actions'. These performances happen naturally in everyday life and the emphasis is on the 'particular'. In this case, the situative performance that interested me was observing home hospice care. The research took place in the emerging palliative care and hospice setting in Ethiopia, which is a 'foreign' setting where perhaps conventional ethnography would be the methodological choice (O'Reilly, 2009). However, my focus was on caring for the dying who are receiving palliative care and a focused ethnography seemed more appropriate. The next part of this chapter will describe the first stumbling block I came across in my research, which was gaining entry to the research site. I will describe the various strategies and skills that I used to gain access. I use extracts from my research diary, which recorded the interactions between various gatekeepers to illustrate the communication and negotiation skills needed to gain entry.

Gaining Entry

Negotiating and gaining entry and access to the research field has been described as a 'balancing act' (Hammersley & Atkinson, 2007, p. 58). In this instance, the balancing act consisted of trying to find the right people at the right time who were able to grant access within the time constraints of my study. To improve the outcome of this balancing act, I used various strategies to assist communication with gatekeepers. The first strategy employed was the use of letters of introduction. My supervisor provided letters of support to help navigate between the officials whom I would need permission from and the organisations I hoped to enter. The letters were on university headed note paper and were stamped with a university stamp. Without an official stamp, no document is seen as genuine in Addis Ababa, as there is a concern that documents can be forged and a stamp is a sign of legitimacy (Blunt, 2009). To support the letters of introduction, I had a one-page summary of my proposed study, which I could use to discuss with key contacts. Another important aspect of preparation was the production of business cards. Business cards are an important part of business etiquette which, in Ethiopia as in Japan, are treated with respect. In Ethiopia, a business card is given and received using the right hand (King, 2013). Business cards turned out to be an invaluable form of introduction for gatekeepers along with the stamped letter from the university.

The gatekeepers that I needed to negotiate with were from three different organisations, namely the hospice organisation where I wanted to conduct my study, the Federal Ministry of Health and the Ethics approval body in Addis Ababa. Identifying relevant gatekeepers is not always easy or straightforward (Hammersley & Atkinson, 2007). Each gatekeeper I went to see subsequently informed me of the next process I would require; for example, the hospice director led me to the Ministry of Health and so on. I encountered the first gatekeeper when deciding on the focus for the study. I needed to get permission to interview and observe, staff, patients and family members who accessed palliative care services. I met with the Director of the Hospice and she granted permission to carry out observations in the hospice. I then discussed the ethical process for research with her. I had already received ethical approval from the University of Surrey, but I also required ethical approval in Ethiopia. She suggested that I should visit the Ministry of Health to ask the director for his advice regarding the ethical process. The hospice director offered to write a letter confirming permission for the study. With the letter from the hospice director and a letter of introduction from the University of Surrey, I then went to the Ministry of Health. After multiple visits, I managed to find the person I needed to see, the Director of the Medical Directorate, and was given an audience. After discussing my research project, he wrote a letter to the organisation, the Ethiopian Health and Nutrition Institute who would consider my documentation for ethical approval. I subsequently spoke to the Head of Ethics. He was very kind and surprised me by guiding me through the process I would need to complete which would involve a protocol and video presentation. This description appears to be a straightforward linear process. However, excerpts from my research diary below illustrate the intricacy and complexity of the emotions involved.

> Waiting at the Ministry of Health…
>
> I sat there waiting, waiting, on a chair beside the secretary's desk at the entrance to a large open plan office. Watching people coming and going. To the left of the desk was an enclosed office that appeared to be the director's office. I have in my hand the letter from the university and the letter from the hospice. I am feeling nervous, as if I am not able to see the director, I don't know if this research is possible. I am sitting here, trying not to look inpatient! I wait for 50 minutes and finally the secretary tells me the director is not available today and she tells me to come back tomorrow.
>
> The next day….

I walk back into the office, the secretary greets me in Amharic and smiles and tells me that she remembers me. So, I am back, sitting on the same chair, anxious again. After about 15 minutes a well-dressed man comes in and walks into the director's office. I continue to sit... the secretary then walks in to speak to him and finally she calls me. I walk in to the office and I think to myself- which language shall I use. I decide in a split second and greet the director warmly in Amharic, using the polite form of the language that is used for an older or important person. He uses the same language form to me. We shake hands. The director is surprised that I am able to speak Amharic and smiles. He then asks me to sit down. I hand over the letters which he studies carefully. He asks me about the university I am studying at. When he sees the letter from the hospice, he smiles, and says 'I know the lady who runs this… she is trying very hard with palliative care'. After seeing the letter from the hospice, the director appeared more relaxed. I asked him about how to get ethical clearance. He explained the different options to me and then offered to write me a letter of introduction to the organisation I would need to work with. During the conversation, I speak in Amharic as much as I am able as I noticed that at the beginning of the conversation it opened the door for dialogue.

Using the description from the research diary of the communication I had at the Ministry of Health with the secretary and the director, I will now discuss my use of reflexivity in more depth.

First, I will consider the importance of reflexivity, and I will also describe the emotions involved, and how reflexivity and emotions intersected for me. Ethnography is driven by the experience of the writer drawing on their work in the field in their area of study, and then interpreting it; in order to do this, the researcher must be reflexive. Reflexivity is a key characteristic of ethnography (Cruz & Higginbottom, 2013) and is a commonly used term with many meanings and little clear understanding (Atkinson & Coffey, 2002). Reflexivity according to Hammersley and Atkinson (2007, p. 15) is shaped by the researcher, their background and interests:

Acknowledges that the orientations of researchers will be shaped by their sociohistorical locations, including the values and interests that these locations confer upon them. What this represents is a rejection of the idea that social research is, or can be, carried out in some autonomous realm that is

> insulated from the biography of the researcher, in such a way that its findings can be unaffected by social processes and personal characteristics.

However, having a meaningful definition of what reflexivity is does not necessarily explain how it is done. Pillow (2003) suggests that reflexivity can be used through the research process, to establish integrity and ensure transparency and validity. Several writers have identified different types of reflexivity and where they occur in the research process (Clifford & Marcus, 1986; Denzin, 1997; Finlay, 2002). To discuss reflexivity with regards to this study, I used Pillow's (2003) four reflexive strategies: 'reflexivity as recognition of self, reflexivity as recognition of other, reflexivity as truth and reflexivity as transcendence' (Pillow, 2003, p. 18). The research diary extracts, illustrate reflexivity as a recognition of self in a situation which was uncomfortable but also a recognition of other in that I was able to not disturb sensibilities by saying the wrong words or behaving in a culturally inappropriate way with key gatekeepers and potential supporters of the research. The premise that it is impossible to be neutral or passive is essential to grasp; that it is the 'sense of self' that affects one's listening and discourse with the participant (Gubrium, Holstein, Marvasti, & McKinney, 2012). Because of this, the importance of critically analysing oneself as a researcher, as well as the research, should not be underestimated (Carolan, 2003). In the extracts from my research diary, you can sense the frustration of waiting at the office to speak to the director! I was frustrated by the waiting and I was also nervous—not a great combination when I am attempting to research a culture where the concept of time is different and where people are treated as more important than time (Hofstede, 1991). I was very nervous about this meeting as the success of my research rested on it. If this gatekeeper was unwilling or unable to assist the process of ethical permission, my study was not going to get off the ground. Nevertheless, my research diary extract also shows I was aware that I must not appear to be impatient. I had to do emotional labour on myself to remain calm, courteous and patient. In this reflection, I see reflexivity as a recognition of self and culture, where my Western understanding of time is different to that of the host culture where people are more important than time. This was essential understanding that I needed to work with to not become impatient and to be critically aware of myself in another culture where different rules apply.

Finding the right place and getting permissions can sometimes be a difficult and an intricate process especially wherever one is working. The problem of where to locate oneself is a major issue when it comes to ethnographic research and Wolcott suggests that serendipity has a lot to do with finding permission for a research project (Wolcott, 1999, p. 24). The serendipity that Wolcott describes is evident during the first visit to the Ministry of Health that appears to have gone nowhere. Actually, it becomes clear at the beginning of the second visit that the waiting involved in the first visit has laid the ground for the second visit, as the secretary greets me in the local language and remembers me. The secretary appears to be the guardian of the gatekeeper, so by spending time waiting patiently the first time around, she seemed to be prepared to speak on my behalf on the second visit. Her willingness to support me enabled the positive interaction with the director and his help in how to go about gaining ethical permission for the study.

The second part of the research diary demonstrates how reflexivity and emotions intersect. Again, I am back at the director's office; however, this time the director is present. I have to make a decision about which language to use. As the director is a doctor, he would speak English as this is the language used to teach at medical college. I decide to speak in Amharic and this sets the scene for the conversation. By using Amharic when you greet someone, it is not a matter of just saying 'hello'; an Amharic greeting includes asking if they are well, if they have peace, about their work, their family. Greetings are essential and intricate in the Amharic language. By using the polite form of the language, I was showing respect to the director, which he in turn showed to me by using the same form. This process is similar to Li's concept of 'symbiotic niceness', where she suggests that nurses' talk functions to preserve a nice, friendly, informal and pleasant atmosphere in interaction' (Li, 2004, p. 2580). In her study, Li identified analytic categories of symbiotic niceness where being mutually nice smoothes communication. The director and myself start the communication by being 'nice'; this then creates an atmosphere where positive communication flows. The director continues the conversation by asking about the university I am studying at, and the conversation deepens when common ground is found by us both knowing the hospice director. I observed that the director appeared to relax when he saw the letter from the hospice. Again, symbiotic niceness is enacted as the director offers words of encouragement and as he comments about the good work of the hospice. One of Li's (2004) categories is 'institutional niceness', whereby a team collectively practises niceness. In the above extract, the director at the Ministry is being nice about another institution 'the hospice'. So both the greetings and the letter from the hospice allowed the director to feel comfortable; he was then happy to help further. The second diary extract demonstrates how using niceness as a communication strategy is helpful in opening doors when trying to gain access. It also shows how important it is to be reflexive in the recognition of self (Pillow, 2003) and to handle immediate emotions, such as frustration and anxiety, through doing emotion work on the self in order to facilitate meaningful communication. The next part of this chapter discusses reflexivity again by looking at the insider/outsider aspects of being a researcher.

Walking the Insider/Outsider Tightrope

Prior to starting the fieldwork, it was important to reflect personally on two essential concepts related to 'self'. First, as a person, what was I bringing to the field? As I am neither neutral nor passive, I needed to reflect on my identities and the effect they would have during the study (Fetterman, 2009). Second, I needed to consider what role I was going to take regarding participant observation. In ethnographic fieldwork, self has been described as the primary research instrument (Wolcott, 1999). That being the case, a self-critical stance was essential to my mind (Silverman, 2013). It is important to locate oneself in the study openly and honestly (O'Reilly, 2009). The ethnographer's role is to understand the social and cultural scene from the insider's (emic) perspective in order to make sense of the data from an outsider's (etic) or 'external social scientific perspective' (Fetterman, 2009). Coffey (1999) suggests that ethnographers are to be 'reflective insiders, negotiating roles and subjectivities, looking out'.

As I started my fieldwork my multiple identities (Coffey, 1999, p. 57) and the awareness I had regarding these identities in the field came to the fore. My supervisors helped me unpack my various identities during our meetings; they helped me think about 'how I came across' and how that would affect my data. My ethnicity as a white woman made me an outsider in a field researching black Ethiopian participants. Although speaking Amharic would provide some insider perspective, as a non-native speaker, I will always be an outsider. With my professional identity as a nurse working in non-governmental organisation relief and development work, with palliative care experience in Yemen and the UK, I had some insider knowledge. Nevertheless, nursing in Ethiopia was a complete unknown. My religious identity as a Protestant Christian would potentially offer some insider perspective as, in Ethiopia, having a faith is an important part of a person's identity. However, to a Muslim participant or an Ethiopian Orthodox Christian, I would again be regarded as an outsider. As a researcher, I would be an obvious outsider. Being female offered both insider/outsider status, as the majority of patients, due to the epidemiology of cancer in Ethiopia, are female. Yet, the majority of gatekeepers, apart from the hospice director, were male. My multiple identities, seemed clear at the beginning of my study. However, getting to that position requires thought, reflection and supportive supervision.

Being aware of self in your research is essential, as it promotes reflexivity. Finlay (2002), like Pillow (2003) identifies multiple categories of reflexivity, one being 'reflexivity as intersubjective reflexion' (Finlay, 2002, p. 215). This is where researchers explore mutual meanings within the research relationship. She argues that there are unconscious processes that structure relationships primarily between the researcher and the participant. An example of this can be seen in the fieldnote extract:

> I was talking with one of the hospice nurses and the father of a little girl who had leukaemia, and who was staying at the hospice whilst she was receiving chemotherapy at the oncology centre. The father was younger than me, so I used the grammatical verb of greeting in Amharic that is used amongst people who are of the same standing. Wondwesen, the hospice nurse, was upset with the way I spoke and told me: 'You can't speak to him like that, he is a priest'. I was so embarrassed and apologised profusely, as I

> was not aware of his standing in the community. The father then smiled and blessed me… this cultural mistake subsequently opened the door for me to talk with him about his daughter. (Field notes)

In the above extract, I am using Amharic to speak to the girl's father and Wondwesen, so there is degree of insider status on my part. Wondwesen and I are both nurses, so again there is a degree of insider status and we are both speaking to a Father. However, Wondwesen is an Ethiopian Orthodox Christian, and the fact that I am speaking to the girl's father who was a priest using familiar language, makes him react, as this was culturally inappropriate and reveals my outsider status as a Protestant Christian who was unaware that the girl's father was a priest. The girl's father was wearing normal country dress, a gabi which is like a large cotton shawl that farmers wear to keep warm. There was no visual cue to me that the girl's father was a priest (often in the city, priests wear a head dress or coloured clothes). There I was in the role of nurse/researcher and the girl's father was in the role of father/priest, and I was completely unaware of his professional capacity. However, the irony of the situation is that the girl's father showed me kindness and blessed me, and my mistake inadvertently opened a dialogue to discuss his daughter's difficult situation. Finlay (2002) calls this 'negotiating the swamp' when the researcher has to navigate the swamp of 'interminable deconstructions, self-analysis and self-disclosure' (Finlay, 2002, p. 209). I felt uncomfortable making such a cultural mistake in front of the girl's father, nevertheless I also had the experience of creating rapport with someone, even though it was from making a mistake. I seemed at this point to understand the muddy waters of reflexivity as intersubjective reflection (Finlay, 2002).

The multiple identities taken and given illustrate the tight-rope of managing insider-outsider status and the emotions experienced by the researcher. By being continually reflexive, it is possible to gain insight into the focus of the research. Throughout my fieldwork, I used field notes and a research diary to document my role as an ethnographer (Wolcott, 1999). I found my fieldwork to be an intriguing, challenging but enjoyable time, where I used my multiple identities and roles to develop relationships, which were key to my research and my subsequent career (Coffey, 1999). However, I would agree with Fetterman (2009) who argues that ethnography is not an orderly process. He suggests that to reach a destination in ethnography, 'it often means taking false paths, coming up against dead ends or detours and sometimes losing the way altogether' (Fetterman, 2009, p. ix).

Blurring Roles as a Researcher

The final stumbling block I am going to discuss here is when roles can become blurred. Previously, I discussed the importance of identifying and being aware of the multiple identities that a researcher brings to a study. However, I found working overseas with vulnerable patients a real challenge. As an ethnographer, creating rapport is imperative to the research process (Fetterman, 2009), as ethnography is built on 'mutually trusting relationships', where being open, friendly and communicative helps with trust (O'Reilly, 2009, p. 175). Strategies of creating rapport can include greetings, sharing food, adopting cultural habits and taking a genuine interest and concern about people. Nevertheless, there is a danger that over rapport and blurring in one's identity and role could be problematic (Watts, 2008). When this happens, the researcher can become too involved in the community they are studying and lose objectivity and distance (Hammersley & Atkinson, 2007). This loss of objectivity can occur at home or overseas; being overseas with less support, can make the researcher more susceptible in this situation.

During the first part of my fieldwork experience, after being accepted by the staff, and being aware of the routines and the running of the hospice, I found that I struggled with balancing insider and outsider identities. There was a point, when I became over involved with the hospice, that I identified myself more as a hospice worker than as a researcher. This was partly due to working in the field alone with participants who were so very ill; sometimes in very desperate circumstances which had an impact emotionally. Hammersley and Atkinson (2007, p. 94) argue that when undertaking field research, ethnographers 'do not always leave the field physically and emotionally unscathed, and they rarely leave unaffected by the experience of the research'. This definitely resonated with my research experience. However, Coffey (1999, p. 100) suggests that fieldwork is meaningful and works because 'we have a physical and emotional presence in the field'. So that field relations are both an opportunity and a risk. I became aware of the over-rapport and blurring of my researcher role, and this was also pointed out to me by my academic supervisors. I think one of the reasons for this happening was that I had worked hard at creating rapport in the beginning but perhaps had not had been as aware of the need to preserve my identity as a researcher. It is interesting to note that Coffey suggests that 'the pursuit of cultural understanding and the process of personal development are intimately rather than tangentially related' (Coffey, 1999, p. 23). To counterbalance this problem, I ensured that I maintained an awareness of my researcher role and developed a way of being more reflexive and analytical about what I was observing to deal with the insider and outsider tension I was experiencing. I did this through writing, journaling, having regular supervision and emailing supportive friends. I found that working through this process helped me to engage ultimately in a more meaningful way with the field and deepened my understanding.

The other thing I noticed during this time was that in my journaling and writing, I became aware of avoiding using evaluating words (Emerson et al., 2011), which helped me to adopt the reflexive stance more fully. O'Reilly (2009, p. 90) suggests that 'it is the balancing of stranger and insider, of taking part and writing about it, that it is the essential nature of ethnography'. Using the strategies described helped me to continue my study with a more balanced approach to my role as observer as participant. An example of dealing with an emotional situation and overcoming the blurring and still keeping my researcher role is illustrated by Danzo's story. I met the same lady with HIV every week as she came to the hospice as a day care patient. Danzo had been on anti-retroviral drugs for five years, and had been keeping well. In the last month of my fieldwork, she suddenly got diarrhoea, she was admitted to the hospice and, after trying multiple treatments, Danzo suddenly died. This was a shock to the staff and the other day care patients. Later, sitting in the office with one of the hospice staff as he wept was extremely hard, and yet I felt that it was inappropriate to leave. I was also upset to hear that Danzo had died. However, after I had processed my own emotions, engaging with the staff and patients helped me understand the situation in a deeper way. I was able to understand that the hospice staff felt that it was wrong that Danzo had died from an opportunistic infection. The staff felt that, if they had been involved earlier, they might have been able to help Danzo. Coffey (1999, p. 159), when discussing emotions in fieldwork, suggests that 'having no emotional connection to the research endeavour, setting or people is indicative of a poorly executed project'. Watts (2008) also argues that when working with vulnerable patients there is a potential for emotional distress from all parties, however this does not have to cause harm but the process itself can lead to benefits for the researcher and the participants. Sitting in the office with the hospice staff allowed me to understand the frustration that the hospice worker felt at not being able to help Danzo. After the hospice worker's (Danny) emotional outburst, he then called the staff and patients together to discuss the situation and encouraged the patients that if they ever got a fever or diarrhoea or other symptoms to call the hospice straightaway. By doing this, Danny offered emotional encouragement in the form of emotional labour. Hochschild (2012) examined how feelings have become commercialised in different workplaces and describes how the workforce uses the construct of 'emotional labour' to 'induce or suppress feeling in order to sustain the outward countenance that produces the proper state of mind in others' (Hochschild, 2012, p. 7). Hochschild also suggests that emotional labour takes place in everyday relationships, which she named emotion work. Danny was upset and frustrated, yet as a carer he supressed his own feelings and was able to encourage the staff and patients with clear instructions so that this situation might be avoided in the future. I also had to do emotion work on myself to supress my feelings in order to observe the frustration that Danny felt when he was in his office. I was then able to investigate the emotional dynamic happening around me.

Being in that situation with Danny and watching him handle and process Danzo's death, helped me see as a researcher the need to tell the story, but yet not to be emotionally passive. Watts (2008, p. 8) argues that with highly sensitive research, unless there is a 'shared emotional space that offers the possibility of trust, a shared narrative space may be difficult to establish'. Watts (2008) further argues that authentication comes by understanding the data through emotional exchanges between the researcher and participants. So, what did I learn personally from this experience? It is possible to over identify with participants as rapport is developed and there is a blurring of identity and role. This is something that needs to be observed through journaling and making field notes. Furthermore, my supervisors played a key role in supporting and helping me identify where I was struggling and where I had slipped into the complete participant role (Junker, 1960). However, it is also paramount to not be emotionally passive or so detached that it does not allow for the creation of a shared emotional space between the researcher and the participant.

Strategies for Reflexivity When Conducting Research in a Different Culture

- When planning to work overseas find out what methods of communication help gain entry to research sites.
- Establish a link with a cultural informant who can advise on cultural aspects of communication.
- Discuss with your supervisor the experiences of being overseas to monitor how identities change as the research progresses.
- Make sure when working overseas that you have regular supervision, this can be through email, phone calls or Skype depending on the country you are working in.
- If working with vulnerable participants, ensure that you have emotional support for yourself.
- Do not be in the field for too long. I split my fieldwork into two parts each three to four months. Discuss this with your supervisor.

Conclusion

Researching overseas needs planning, cultural awareness, reflexivity and good supervision. Reading relevant texts whilst planning to research overseas is also very helpful. Thinking about what you and your background bring to the research and reflecting on the multiple identities that emerge are important. Having a cultural informant to discuss issues in your research, especially communication and cultural differences as they arise is important. Furthermore, I would also suggest that the length of fieldwork is considered carefully and make sure that you have adequate support, especially when researching vulnerable groups. Researching overseas can be fun and rewarding and lessons can be learnt from experiencing different cultures, but reflexivity is the passport to success.

References

Atkinson, P., & Coffey, A. (2002). Revisiting the relationship between participant observation and interviewing. In J. F. Gubrium & J. A. Holstein (Eds.), *Handbook of interview research*. Thousand Oaks, CA: Sage.

Blunt, E. (2009). *Ethiopia's passion for bureaucracy*. Retrieved August 16, 2013, from http://news.bbc.co.uk/1/hi/8189145.stm

Carolan, M. (2003). Reflexivity: A personal journey during data collection. *Nurse Researcher, 10*(3), 7–14. https://doi.org/10.7748/nr2003.04.10.3.7.c5892

Clifford, J., & Marcus, G. (1986). *Writing culture: The poetry and politics of ethnography* (25th Anniversary ed.). California: University of California Press.

Coffey, A. (1999). *The ethnographic self: Fieldwork and the representation of identity* (1st ed.). London: Sage.

Cruz, E. V., & Higginbottom, G. (2013). The use of focused ethnography in nursing research. *Nurse Researcher, 20*(4), 36–43.

Denzin, N. (1997). *Interpretive ethnography: Ethnographic practices for the 21st century*. Thousand Oaks, CA: Sage.

Fetterman, D. (2009). *Ethnography: Step by step* (3rd ed.). London: Sage.

Finlay, L. (2002). Negotiating the swamp: The opportunity and challenge of reflexivity in research practice. *Qualitative Research, 2*(209), 209–230.

Gubrium, J. F., Holstein, J., Marvasti, A. B., & McKinney, K. D. (Eds.). (2012). *The SAGE handbook of interview research: The complexity of the craft* (2nd ed.). Thousand Oaks, CA: Sage.

Hammersley, M., & Atkinson, P. (2007). *Ethnography principles in practice* (3rd ed.). Abingdon: Routledge.

Hochschild, A. R. (2012). *The Managed heart commercialization of human feeling* (1st revised ed.). California: University of California Press.

Hofstede, G. H. (1991). *Cultures and organisations software of the mind* (2nd ed.). London: McGraw-Hill International.

King, T. (2013). *Business etiquette in global business scenarios*. Retrieved August 16, 2013, from http://www.ehow.com/about6514742_business-etiquette-global-business-scenarios.html
Knoblauch, H. (2005). Focused ethnography. *Forum: Qualitative Social Research, 6*(3), 1–13.
Li, S. (2004). Symbiotic niceness: Constructing a therapeutic relationship in psychosocial care. *Social Science and Medicine, 58*, 2571–2583.
O'Reilly, K. (2009). *Key concepts in ethnography*. London: Sage.
Pillow, W. (2003). Confession, catharsis, or cure? Rethinking the uses of reflexivity as methodological power in qualitative research. *Qualitative Studies in Education, 16*(2), 175–196.
Seale, C. (1998). *Constructing death: The sociology of dying and bereavement*. Cambridge: Cambridge University Press.
Silverman, D. (2013). *Doing qualitative research* (4th ed.). London: Sage.
Walter, T. (1994). *The revival of death*. London: Routledge.
Watts, J. H. (2008). Emotion, empathy and exit: Reflections on doing ethnographic qualitative research on sensitive topics. *Medical Sociology Online, 3*(2), 3–14.
Wolcott, H. F. (1999). *Ethnography. A way of seeing*. Walnut Creek, CA: AltaMira Press.

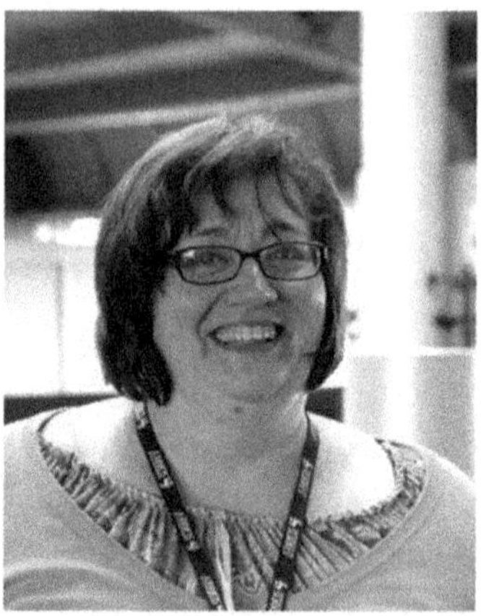

Nicola Ayers is a Palliative Care Advisor at the Clinical Services Directorate, Federal Ministry of Health, Ethiopia. She was awarded her Ph.D. from the University of Surrey in 2015.

8

Emotion Work in Ethnography

Ginny Mounce

Introduction

In this chapter, I explore the impact of emotion work on my research, including how questions of risk, reactivity and privacy were resolved. My thesis concerned the experiences of infertile and sub-fertile couples who were starting fertility treatments. The nature of the study meant that I collected sensitive, highly emotional and intimate data. This presented me with challenges during fieldwork, including how I collected data from participants and how I maintained relationships with participants in the light of the information shared with me. The knowledge that I was likely to stir up unwelcome feelings in both myself and others, to encounter grief and to possibly cause anguish was a form of emotional risk. There was the potential for 'emotional danger', that is, threatening and negative feelings experienced by myself and the participants (Lee-Treweek & Linkogle, 2000).

G. Mounce (✉)
Nuffield Department of Obstetrics and Gynaecology, University of Oxford, Oxford, UK

H.T. Allan, A. Arber (eds.), *Emotions and reflexivity in Health and Social Care Field Research*, https://doi.org/10.1007/978-3-319-65503-1_8

To investigate the lived experiences of couples, I had designed a longitudinal ethnographic study which used observations in the clinic and repeat interviews. In common with other longitudinal work, the data collection period was long—amounting to eighteen months in the field—with multiple data collection points. Knowledge about the social reality under investigation is formed by the social interactions of the researcher and the researched, which gives rise to field relationships developed over time and shaped by the stance of the researcher (Allen, 2004). Other contributors have written about insider-outsider roles. In this chapter, the focus is on *reactivity* (Hammersley, 2013; Pelto, 2016) by which I mean the effect of the researcher on the field and its participants who may or may not be participants in the research but who inhabit the field. Accordingly, the reflexivity which I employed was the variant Finlay called 'intersubjective', that is, concerned with the mutual meanings of the shared field relationship (Finlay, 2002a). When I wrote my research proposal, I had the idea that the ethnographic tension of reactivity might be reduced by greater familiarity between myself and my participants, that repeat interviews might be empowering, for participants and for myself. I also wondered if the research encounters would become easier as the relationship between us developed. However, I found the sustained involvement with the participants in this design brought with it other tensions.

I thought that to research emotion work would be similar to my midwifery experience (Hunter, 2001). It seemed to me that research in highly sensitive areas which necessitated developing 'empathetic distance' with participants (Rowling, 1999) is similar to debates about emotion management in midwifery (Hunter, 2001). Would I express empathy and caring differently in a research relationship? When I considered privacy before entering the field, I wondered: how I would access their private accounts of experiences or certain things which could not be said by participants or questions which I could not ask? I did not consider the effect of such private accounts being disclosed through my relationship with participants or the effect on me personally at an emotional level. During interviews, I asked the couples to articulate and reveal their innermost thoughts and feelings about infertility, and I sometimes observed them during the intimacy of the clinic procedures. What follows is a consideration of all these issues in greater detail.

Locating the Self in the Research

As I was engaged in phenomenological research, I understood myself as integral to the social world I studied and located myself accordingly within the research (Finlay, 2002b; Lipson, 1991). Phenomenology takes the subjective perspective as its empirical starting point (Van Manen, 1990). However, gaining an understanding of another's subjective experience is a complex undertaking which is possible only through interpretation. As researchers we exist, 'being-in-the-world' ourselves and are unable to be detached observers; our understanding of phenomena is always based on our background and the historicality of our past experience in the world, whether consciously experienced or not (Koch, 1996). I used participant observation and interviews to collect data and facilitate the emic, insider view but the sense and meanings of participants' experiences were filtered through my understandings (Porter, 2000). Reflexivity is the explicit recognition of this, the process by which I, as researcher, acknowledged my place in the research.

In ethnography, reflexive practice is encouraged by the use of diaries and fieldnotes as they provide a means of critical self-reflection on events and a space for recording emotions, thoughts and accounts of tensions that arise during the research process (Coffey, 1999). Maintaining a balanced insider-outsider relationship has always been a concern of ethnographic method, often referred to as 'keeping the familiar strange and the strange familiar' (Hammersley & Atkinson, 2007, p. 231). Having a reflexive attitude through contemplating their role in a research study is one way the researcher can achieve this. With this, ethnographers have always been committed to seeing the social world from the viewpoint of the subject, (Bryman, 1984) and much ethnographic fieldwork is concerned with obtaining access to the social lives of insiders.[1] Ethnography privileges the position of the researcher through the power they have in representing their participants to the 'outside' (Pillow, 2003). Reflexivity is employed to unmask this: to show that participants are not only telling stories but the stories that the researcher wants to hear.

The literature on reflexivity, even that critical of its practice (Pillow, 2003), suggests that actually 'doing reflexivity' or being a reflexive practitioner is not something which can be easily taught (Finlay, 2008). It is not simply a case of thinking reflectively about an event or moment, but an active process of being aware of oneself as 'other' and being able to locate oneself in the research. The researcher is the conduit of the research: choosing the questions to ask or avoid and interpreting the data, deciding what is noted and recorded, deciding how questions are framed, what meanings are attached to things that are said or done, and understandings of each and so on. Consequently, I understood that my research would be uniquely mine. My responsibility was not only to give voice to my participants, but also to make my own perspectives, biases and leanings aware to the readers of my outputs. However, as I suggested earlier, this is itself problematic for, as Pillow says, even the notion of 'giving voice' to participants already privileges the superior, knowing voice of the researcher (Pillow, 2003); something which a postmodernist ethnographer attempts to avoid.

The concern of postmodern ethnography is with truth claims and other representations associated with traditional ethnography (Fontana, 2004; Williams, 1990). Today, researchers widen their reflexivity to show, as I have done, their decision-making and how the research was done. In rejecting the idea that a single authoritative voice can provide an explanation for the data, a postmodern ethnographer attempts to disclose the multiple meanings and voices associated with the phenomenon and the representation of the phenomenon (Brewer, 2000). Another goal, again rejecting the idea of 'neutrality' in representation, is for research findings to be understood in terms of the culture being studied and attending to issues of gender relations or power.

Although I identify as a novice researcher with little previous experience of qualitative methodologies I had hoped that being a midwife would be helpful towards my reflexivity, as 'reflective practice' is a common, increasingly mandatory, exercise for appraisal and learning in my profession (Collington & Hunt, 2006). Therefore, some of the ideas of critical analysis, evaluation and self-awareness which this entails (Finlay, 2008) were already familiar to me from processes including annual supervision and practice development. I was less familiar with reflexivity in research practice. Furthermore, the type of reflection dominant in nursing and midwifery practice tends to be a kind of introspective 'thinking about' something, and lacks wider theoretical focus (Finlay, 2008). The concept of reflexion exists at the other end of a continuum to this simple sort of 'reflection'; reflexion is immediate conscious self-awareness which includes the social contexts of actions (Finlay, 2002b).

A key aspect of being a reflective practitioner or researcher therefore is of 'being in the moment', that is, being able to simultaneously reflect on what is happening (experience) while remaining engaged with whatever the encounter is (Schön, 1983). Whether this is even feasible is debatable as, for example, not all phenomenologists accept that it is possible to split the mind, actions and emotions in this manner because of the embodiment of being-in-the-world. For practical purposes though, it is argued that reflection and action can occur *more or less* simultaneously with practice (Finlay, 2008). In practice, I was uneasily aware of myself in my various roles as both a researcher and a clinic insider (Pellatt, 2003); I was preoccupied with how I positioned myself, what I was wearing, how I should take notes and what other people, both staff colleagues and participants, thought of what I was doing. The participants appeared to be unquestioning of what I was or was not doing in both my observation and participatory roles. Instead it was I who became anxious when research participants confused my research role by asking me questions in consultations or caught my eye (although the doctors did this too during my observations of medical consultations). I was much more focussed and aware of myself being in the clinic than they were. For example, in consultations I consciously kept my head down and moved my chair out of their eye line (in case they tried to include me). And in interviews with participants, I switched the tape recorder off when they wanted advice or wanted me to discuss clinical matters with them. Looking back, I can see that while I was still trying to work out what my research role and stance should be. I was probably overly concerned with establishing distance (Rowling, 1999). One of Rowling's participants admitted they 'hadn't thought about' her role in the research encounter, beyond it being 'professional', and I suspect this would have been similar in my situation. In other words, the boundary between my research and clinical roles was blurred, but seemingly this was of little importance to the participants or other actors in the clinic.

On occasion, participants asked my insider opinion or for my help in sorting out issues they had with the fertility clinic. One example included Cath[2] who phoned me after her first consultation with a doctor to tell me how unhappy she had been with it. She asked for my advice about what to do. I organised for Cath and her partner Andy to have another appointment, this time with a more senior doctor. Afterwards I was worried that this action would have somehow contaminated my data as it had changed their experience of what the encounter at the clinic had been. With more thought, I reasoned that what I had done was not that unusual as it was merely a normal social interaction, and it is not uncommon in healthcare practice for things to work like this. In the end, I decided that it had given me another perspective on their experience and wrote:

> This is a slightly odd situation as I have now become an insider, and of course this might not have been dealt with in the same way if she hadn't known me. Although actually if she had phoned the clinic I think they would have given her a new appointment, maybe not as quickly!

In a later telephone call, Cath and I discussed some of the concerns she had raised with the clinic manager about this first appointment. Together we decided to postpone our research interview until after the rearranged consultation for the reason that 'otherwise she's going to be spending her whole time complaining about the consultation'. In hindsight, this was a missed opportunity as an interview would have given me further insights into what they were feeling. In the end, the second consultation was also enlightening; I felt I'd gained an insider's perspective of the matters which were of most importance to them *and* an awareness of the attitude the clinic staff had towards this couple, as I noted:

> Later the administrator starts getting quite irritated with this couple because now they've been asking her more questions! How dare they! It seems they have reached their 'quota' of allocated time and attention and should just be grateful for what they've been given (despite the fact that their consultation wasn't up to par)

As the following examples show there were several other occasions, particularly at the beginning of my fieldwork, where it seems clear that I was negotiating my identity as researcher at the clinic. Part of this was because some of the nursing staff questioned my new role in the clinic:

> One of the nurses saw me later that afternoon and said 'what are you doing sitting in the waiting room with your pad and clip board today?' So I told her I was doing a study which involved me observing and interviewing people and she said she hoped 'I wasn't observing her doing something wrong' as she felt "quite nervous". All this was said in a jokey manner and I don't think this is a problem as this particular nurse is quite inquisitive and approves of and takes an interest in my studying.

The doctors were curious about what I was doing, but only because they associated observation with audit and assessment. They all questioned me and were concerned with what it meant for them. The most senior consultant asked me 'did I pass?' Another made a joke when I first asked him if I could sit in on his consultation:

> He said "no!" and then, at my startled reaction, gleefully told me how he likes to give people unexpected answers to questions because [he likes to see] their reactions. Quite odd?'

I suspected this doctor was unsettled by my request, and that his peculiar reply was in some way a projection of his own fear of the unknown. His response was unsettling for me too as it was unexpected, and I found this exchange quite uncomfortable. Later I was able to observe a couple of his consultations, and he always requested 'feedback'. Another claimed 'to like it' (being observed) because of the opportunity it gave for their own learning. The clinicians all equated observation with practice rather than research. Another asked me if I thought he'd been too harsh to the couple because she'd become upset. I told him the purpose of my being there was not to make judgements about him and how he was conducting his consultation, that I was observing the couples. Later, on reflection, I wondered if I had missed a good opportunity to talk to him about this. After all this is ethnography and would have been a good example of a spontaneous corridor conversation and would have told me something about the culture of the clinic. So I suggested that if he'd like to I'd be really interested to hear his thoughts about any other sessions that I observed with him. He seemed pleased and positive about doing this in the future, especially if they were interesting cases. This remark is quite telling in itself as it demonstrates how routine the consultations are for the clinicians, while my data confirmed that they were extremely important to my participants.

Emotional Risk

Discussing the topic of researcher safety, Lee-Treweek and Linkogle (2000) acknowledge the risks inherent in researching any emotional subject. The threat is from the negative feelings and destabilising state which may be induced from thinking about or hearing accounts that are unsettling and upsetting. The emotional risk inherent in researching sensitive topics is increasingly discussed (Dickson-Swift, James, Kippen, & Liamputtong, 2008), and strategies to minimise such risks, for example, professional supervision and training, have been proposed to counter these. Much of the management of this risk is borne by individuals, who seek an understanding of social realities which have as their defining features emotions and sensitivities. Therefore, this work can be challenging, especially if the topic chimes personally although this was not the case for me. In choosing to research experiences of infertility I was aware that my research participants were often experiencing great hurt and sorrow, akin to grief, and that this would likely arouse uncomfortable feelings for both of us. However, unlike others who have chosen to study this topic (Allan, 1997; Letherby, 2000) I did not identify with my subjects through any immediate personal experience of infertility but I did not view this as a disadvantage.

Letherby argues that she enjoyed greater intimacy and rapport with her respondents as a direct result of her own history (Letherby, 2000). She further suggests that her perceptions and understandings were enhanced because of her commitment and enthusiasm for the topic. Her account illustrates how her own experiences were present in her research, from her choice of topic to interpretation of findings. However, the identity of the researcher as 'other' is complex, and no one identity in the field is privileged. My identity as researcher was multiple; gendered (as a woman), academic, mother, midwife and fertility researcher all gave me different perspectives and connections with my participants. An instant sympathy with and ability to relate to some participants over others, was likely to be the result of a combination of attitudes, interests and experiences, rather than a single common history. Pillow (2003) critiques strategies of self-reflexivity in which coming to 'know oneself', often through confessional tales or finding experiences in common with the research subjects, become a comfortable act that has the effect of making both researcher and researched more familiar to each other, rather than being used to expose the difficulties and differences inherent in knowing the other (Pillow, 2003). In addition, the introspection and self-awareness necessary for reflexivity to be meaningful should not be allowed to take over the focus of the research; reflexion is not all about the researcher per se and, as Finaly (1998) warns, is 'neither an opportunity to wallow in subjectivity nor permission to engage in legitimised emoting' (Finaly, 1998, p. 455). As described earlier, and importantly, reflexion is distinct from reflection because it includes an awareness of 'other', and is not *just* a conscious self-awareness or, in Finlay's words again, 'navel-gazing' (Finlay, 2002a).

The 'swamp' that Finlay describes as the challenge of reflexion is illustrative of its problematic nature (Finlay, 2002a). Phenomenologists are particularly interested in how the 'subject is present in the object' and believe that reflexivity aids in pointing out how differences in our experiences of the same thing are traceable to differences in 'the horizons' through which we experience them (Holloway & Galvin, 2017). My own experiences of reflexivity have been sometimes disconcerting and, as both Finlay (2002a) and Pillow (2003) suggest, 'messy' (Finlay, 2002a; Pillow, 2003). This was because I found it uncomfortable to interrogate my ideas and thoughts; ask questions of myself about why I came to think the way I did or how my understandings of my participants' perspective were realised. It is clear that I used a form of intersubjective reflexivity rather than a broader form of postmodern critique as mentioned earlier (Finlay, 2002a). But as the research developed, my awareness of the broader social critique of care provision for infertile people grew. My main concerns initially were with the relationship between myself and the researched, and in identifying the differences in our situated meanings. I had selected my topic because of its familiarity and interest to me. Currently my day-to-day working life is based in a fertility clinic; it was while I was new to the clinic that I started thinking about the experiences of the people I observed and met there. I had all sorts of thoughts about the various attitudes, behaviours and actions of both staff and patients, and I had my own ideas about why these might be the way they were. The clinic seemed to be a particular world of which I was not quite a part. As a research nurse, I have a dual role, neither completely 'one of them' [the staff] but also somewhat socialised as a clinic insider. I felt that this was a perfect starting point for ethnographic fieldwork and participant observation much as others have (Arber, 2006).

Accessing the distressing feelings of participants was important as a means of identifying closely with their experiences and providing a genuine 'insider' point of view. I found the emotional distancing inherent in the development of a 'working persona' (Mackintosh, 2007), which I had employed as a practising midwife, helpful in relation to this. The emotional labour that midwives do is often a consequence of their presence in highly emotional, often sad, situations (Hunter & Deery, 2009). Therefore, the experience of being with men and women expressing their feelings was not unfamiliar to me, although that is not to say that I had no personal response to it or had become immune to it. Emotion work is skilled work which has to be learnt despite being undervalued for being perceived as natural to women (Hunter, 2001). Clearly social researchers who are not health service professionals also have interactions with their participants like these and are therefore faced with the similar issues of emotional labour (Dickson-Swift, James, Kippen, & Liamputtong, 2009). The management of emotions is not concerned with preserving researcher detachment or neutrality as in positivist research (Watts, 2007) but to protect the researcher and the researched from negative consequences of emotion work, such as depression and anxiety (Dickson-Swift et al., 2009). Strategies of 'self-care' adopted by social researchers to manage their emotions generally involve methods of distancing, for example reminding themselves that 'the research was not about them'. Nevertheless, it is clear that these sorts of strategies are not always easy to adopt in practice and it is sometimes necessary to utilise more formal support strategies. Supervision, or similar structured debriefing, is useful because the analysis it entails can be transformative; positive feelings are generated through problem solving, and the disclosure in supervision is another psychological strategy for coping with negative emotions (McLeod, 2009). I found my own emotional coping methods of distraction, exercise and diary-keeping helpful, similar to the distancing strategies and focus on 'own time' used by nurses in emotionally demanding roles (Froggatt, 1995). Other cognitive techniques such as meditation and mindfulness are also said to be useful for some individuals in this respect (McLeod, 2009).

However, ethnographic fieldwork is concerned with emotions and having reactions of anger, sadness, joy, sorrow and various other feelings was to be expected (Coffey, 1999). My experience of fieldwork was no exception. It is worth stating here that I do not believe emotions should be absent from academic work, even though I, like Watts (2007), am unconvinced that it is always possible to integrate them successfully. Like other researchers, I found that I responded emotionally to some of the things I saw or heard, but usually it was after the research episode that I felt able to release my emotions. I do not think that the emotional management that Hochschild (1983) described was at play here as the empathy I offered my participants was genuine—by which I mean authentic—rather than a socially acceptable and expected behaviour (Watts, 2007). The commercialisation of consumer and market research has informed techniques of interviewing which aim to encourage the disclosure of private thoughts, but these methods were not known to me (Duncombe & Jessop, 2002). Instead empathy arose through identification with the emotions of others my participants (Hedican, 2008), either through shared or relational experience (Jones & Ficklin, 2012). As Watts suggests, empathy promotes feelings of trust and rapport in relationships, and includes non-verbal components such as touch (Watts, 2007). Demonstrating oneself as empathetic is difficult because it often consists of an attitude as much as anything else. Here is an example from part of an interview with Sara which I responded to with empathy:

S: I was drained at the end of all that
Gm: Were you?
S: Yes, I was quite—even though I knew what to expect—because my friend had um [pause] oh, who has got pregnant which is really exciting!

Gm: Oh, gosh, lovely
S: Yes from IVF…my friend went through it all with me
Gm: Oh yeah that's right, you'd said hadn't you
S: And so even though I knew what, exactly what, and I'd read the thing, it's still kinda quite ..if someone says it's you it makes it all kind of 'real' and it's a bit, you know. And there's all the permissions and it's all quite 'heavy' stuff isn't it?
Gm: It is heavy stuff [long pause]

Using empathy here was not because I had experience of or memory of a similar situation myself, but perhaps through experience of being in the clinic as a midwife/researcher. I shared an understanding of aspects of Sara's emotions as an understanding of what problems are like for her 'heavy stuff' a weight to be borne (Hedican, 2008).

Similar to other authors (Dickson-Swift et al., 2008), I found transcribing interviews to be emotional despite having conducted the interviews. I had already experienced the dialogue and reacted in the moment to it. I knew before transcribing what I was going to hear, but experiencing the stories again, being focussed and absorbed by the aural account was emotionally powerful. The physical process of transcribing, which involved me listening on headphones, being immersed in the narratives and hearing the same story recounted over and over again (because of my slow typing skills) often made me very sad:

> Also it's heart-breaking to listen again to the interview while I am typing it. In between the rational comes little bits and pieces of the emotion that is being suppressed (seems very similar to someone grieving or breaking up with someone). On a personal level it's also moving—I want to be able to help their situation, but of course I can't. The desire to offer advice or encouragement or information is almost unbearable.

And similarly:

> This couple are the ones that I find the most moving. Hearing this again makes me remember the feeling I had at the time which was great sadness and an almost overwhelming wish that I could make it alright. I can't.

When I re-read the notes I made after interviewing John and Thea, I can clearly recall the sadness I felt at the time, when I sat in my car after I had interviewed them.

My emotions were sometimes happy as I responded to the changing moods and situations of my participants, for example I was very relieved and happy for Becky and Ali when they had a pregnancy scan that was all fine and struggled to keep my feelings in check:

> Waited until I knew pregnancy scan result and it's ok! I am really, really delighted (and relieved). I saw them in corridor to check if I can arrange another interview. Gave Becky a hug and 'congratulations'. (Very unlike me—don't do hugging!) We are both a bit teary.

This was an example where I feel my role as researcher allowed me to cross over the boundaries of my clinical role, as in practice I very rarely hug patients like this.

Reactivity

As I described previously in the first research encounter, couples both told their story and set the scene. I felt that as time went on couples became more guarded about their feelings and I wondered if this was a protective mechanism; that is, to prevent me from continuously picking away at something which was painful, so the research process may have become increasingly difficult for them and for me. The optimism that many expressed in the first interview was often unrewarded, something which may have led them to become less expansive, and more introspective. My data showed many of them tried to stay in the moment and not look too far ahead. As time went on I felt less able to ask probing and searching questions of my participants. For example, after one partner had given me their perspective on an event and the other was quiet I had wanted to draw them out and ask them 'Okay, what did you feel about this (and why is it different?)', but their reluctance to make their feelings known in public was clear. In this instance, I felt further questioning would be intrusive. Couples were most protective of privacy around their own relationship and as in this case, it was because of the obvious friction between the couple that I had felt unable to probe further. Sometimes individuals told me about their private feelings but less about their differences as couples. It was questions about their relationship which I found most difficult to ask.

Contrary to my hopes that being in the field for a reasonably long period would add to the depth of the data elicited, as our relationships developed into friendships, I was *more* aware of their characters, world-views and sensitivities and was consequently unwilling to disturb the smooth equilibrium of our relationship. Yet the opportunity that repeat interviews gave was the ability for me to revisit subjects with couples, use short-cuts and jokes to signify that I recognised their emotions and, more prosaically, to get clarification about previous statements. I noted for example that Victoria and David were becoming more like friends than research subjects and that we embrace/kiss to greet each other. David became much freer in his conversation; in one of our later interviews for example he was asking about the processes involved in being a sperm donor. When I explained that it took a long time, he quipped was it the 'speed it takes to masturbate or their paperwork? [ha ha!]', something I am sure he would not have said the first times when we knew each other less well. I enjoyed Victoria and David's company but I was not sure how to be a real friend to people with whom I also had a research relationship (Watts, 2007). I was anxious about having to curb our friendship when I left the field and I felt guilty leaving them after, as Maynard (1994) says, 'stirring it all up'. After we had met for the third and final interview I noted that:

> I draw a line under this now. I need to complete this interview. They have been lovely and I wish them every happiness. I hope it works out—in between their two personalities they both seem very loving [to each other]—they are still 'trying' so who knows? David walks me back to my car and says 'I hope we see you again' which is really kind but probably unrealistic, and with the best will in the world 'I hope I don't'. Really sad evening.[3]

As this example demonstrates even those research relationships that include genuine rapport and empathy only really exist for the purpose of providing data for research. This is uncomfortable to acknowledge, but any research friendship is probably temporary, although this becomes blurred with repeated contact. Duncombe and Jessop (2002) described how their experiences of chance encounters with former interviewees, similar to that I have described above, illuminated the extent to which this occurred. Similar to other researchers I had found it easier to develop rapport with participants who shared demographic characteristics with me, or who had lives closer to my own (Duncombe & Jessop, 2002).

Thea was another woman with whom I had a connection and multiple contacts. Earlier I described that I had found her and John's story very touching, but I found myself withdrawing from engagement with them, particularly Thea, because of a fear that I would be overwhelmed by the sadness that contact with them provoked. This was an example of where my own support mechanisms were important for working through my own feelings of vulnerability that the research relationship with Thea had provoked. The dropping of the clinician boundary put me (the researcher) in a vulnerable position and good support became important here. I started to feel the need for distancing and emotion management. Thea came on her own to meet a consultant after a round of medication had not resulted in pregnancy:

> [Thea] is nervous when I get here, 'I don't know why' [she said] and we talked. I said it was 'a bit like a job interview' and that she needs to feel that she'll get something out of it (hence the nerves) which she agrees with. She said she was 'glad to have me there'… I can remember thinking that she seems very vulnerable sitting the other side of the desk to the Consultant today. She knew what he would say and what he was like. I feel a bit let down by John not turning up. I've just come out of the consultation with [Consultant] and Thea and of course she was immediately just crying. Pent up frustration. I have left it up to her again to contact me but she did say it was ok to contact her. She said that in fact it (talking to me) helps and gives her a chance to talk to John. I said I'd give her a call in a month or so. Clearly she was tearful in the consultation. And she's got to fight him as well (I mean John). It was difficult for her that there is nothing left to do, except IVF which I suspect she wants but he doesn't.
>
> [Few weeks later]. I rang Thea as I hadn't heard anything from her since this. No answer. Left an answerphone message. I need to follow up, but clearly I am not looking forward to doing this.

I strongly felt guilty on leaving this research relationship, and I felt as if I had let Thea down. I felt guilt at other times as well:

> Had a voicemail from Victoria tonight which I initially felt reluctant to listen to. I had to steel myself to do so; a mixture of worry that she would be pulling out of the research and slight heart-sink that it would be a long and emotional call. Happily however, when I did listen it was just to tell me that she had been offered a cancellation (for surgery) and so was not a problem call. I feel a bit guilty about this, but mainly relieved. However, it's becoming a little tiring having to worry about these calls.

These sorts of feelings are however only present because of the genuine concern and empathy present in our research relationships, and I hope that in small ways the reliable presence of an interested researcher was some consolation to my participants.

Privacy

Infertility is a stigmatised condition and researching it involves asking participants to discuss areas of their lives that are normally kept private. Medical treatments are of a highly personal nature, but often take place in clinics where procedures are technical and have become routinised. I was surprised at how willing couples were to become my research participants, to discuss these familiar aspects of their lives and to have me witness some of these episodes. Sara and Dev were a couple who I had a lot of contact with. The first time that I met them was when they had a consultation with a doctor while I observed. The doctor asked if a medical student could also be present and they said afterwards:

> I did have this kind of moment where I was thinking 'oh my goodness how many people can we have in the room, and we are talking about our sex life and it's just, but it was very… it was surreal'!

At a subsequent appointment, I observed Sara having a HyCoSy scan, an intimate clinical procedure involving an internal (vaginal) scan, carried out by a nurse. This proved to be a painful and distressing experience for Sara:

> Today Sara is having HyCoSy scan. The waiting room is empty. She is nervous (clearly), laughing nervously. On her own. So I go in (I wasn't planning on doing this, but seems to be the best thing). AB is doing procedure, assisted by a sonographer. I know them both and they both include me in the procedure. Sara tells them that humour is her coping strategy. She takes shoes off and gets ready. The procedure is in an embryo transfer room, essentially a clinic room. Very sterile, bed with stirrups, no soft furnishings etc. I sit next to the bed and try to be inconspicuous (keep out of their way). AB checks Sara has taken pain killers, explains what she is doing etc, Dev is picking Sara up after the procedure. It's her birthday tomorrow, lots of joking about this. Generally, the procedure is clearly very uncomfortable despite Sara's laughter. She says that 'the thought of it is making her tense up'. She talks a lot through it, AB is concentrating hard as the scan and procedure appears tricky, Sara asks if she is 'playing ball' and then says 'it's nothing to do with me, obviously!' also that it's 'a bit crampy'. My impression is that it's a nasty procedure. Sara says it's like 'period pains and really horrible'. Sara says 'you never really know if you are being a wuss' (she's said this before). We all (the other three women) are in agreement that it's a horrible procedure. Sara now says 'if I need you to stop can I just say?', although she then says it's 'just uncomfortable' (trying hard to be brave?) The sonographer says 'if Ginny was any good she'd hold your hand' which I found quite irritating as I was trying to be invisible and make notes! (She wasn't doing anything either). AB is concentrating as she can't see any dye leaving the tubes although they (the tubes) have stopped spasms now. They talk about what was going to be the next step.

Sara and I talked about this event time and time again in subsequent interviews, which emphasised how important this procedure had been for her. I believe I might have missed its significance if I had not observed it or if it had not been for her repeat comments about what she had felt and experienced at the time. Her main focus was on how painful the procedure had been despite the fact that she had convinced herself that the anticipation would have been worse than the event. Being present while someone is in pain is also a part of the emotional labour that midwives do, but I found being an observer troubling. It was clear how the routine of clinic procedures, such as this scan, reinforced the detachment shown by clinical staff to the patient's experience. Sara's eloquence about her experience, and my personal investment in her story, gave me a perspective of this event which I would not otherwise have had.

The reflexion on this event is an example of where the differences in our 'horizons of experience' were brought into relief. Sara's thoughts about and anticipation of the HyCoSy scan were crucial in understanding the meaning the experience had for her. Her statement, such as 'it is the not knowing that is worse', is a standard phrase that, for me, carries little meaning beyond stating you are not looking forward to something. My attitude towards the scan was that it was a routine, predictable event, similar to many other procedures familiar to me in my working life. It was enacted on a body (seemingly unconnected from Sara) and with a known purpose and outcome. For Sara, the experience was fully embodied, painful and frightening, with unknown and unexpected consequences in an environment that was alien to her. Embodiment is the idea that human perceptions and experiences are inseparable from physical and social existence or being-in-the-world (Merleau-Ponty, 1962). The belief that the way the world is experienced by people is through their body (all their bodily senses) and not just through consciousness. Understandings of human experiences therefore must relate to their physical presence in the social and cultural world. Sara's recall of the physicality of the experience reminded me about how casually we health professionals can come to view bodily experience as if, for the other, the mind and body are separate. In the fertility clinic, the (female) body is often investigated through a technological lens which further separates this duality. Frequently, as with Sara's scan, clinical staff in the room are focussed on the screen which shows a picture of her insides, rather than the person on the bed at the centre of the experience. In her description, Sara also verbally separates her cervix from her own self when she asks why the procedure is tricky, and this is not an uncommon experience for infertile women who feel their bodies have let them down (Greil, Slauson-Blevins, & McQuillan, 2010).

The received view of intimacy in relationships and friendship is that individuals are more open with people they are close to and more likely to exchange confidences. The research interview then has an inherent social tension as it breeches social norms in (the UK) society as participants were willing to offer me, a stranger, access to their thoughts and feelings for data collection and analysis. In my notes after the first interview with Thea and John I recognise this tension and the power of the interview and the field relationship:

> This is proper stream of consciousness stuff, and it's heart-breaking, but amazing at the same time.

This comment also reminds me of the importance of participant observation as a source of data in ethnography. Narrative accounts rely on the ability of the participants to articulate their thoughts and experiences (Brocki & Wearden, 2006). I found the first interview I had with all my participants was often the one in which they were most likely to try and express how they felt, and it was then that I was able to ask innocent questions to try and establish their initial thoughts about their experiences. During the first interview with John and Thea, I asked her about her feelings being around other people with babies. I noted that I felt awkward asking this question, but felt I needed to ask it. Although afterwards I was reassured that:

> Actually when Thea laughs and answers this question, she sounds 'relieved'—probably that she can talk about this which, clearly as from what comes afterwards, she needed to talk about.

I reflected further when I followed-up with questions about her feelings of loss:

> I feel a bit sick seeing that I have asked this. It is *so* personal and probing (and obviously I know what the answer is going to be). This is something which I find quite difficult in the interviewing. Sometimes it seems obvious that the couple are not really telling me what they think, but it's quite difficult to get over (my) barrier of asking them the question I need to. I think it's because it's not counselling (and they never signed up for that). However, nobody so far has seemed affronted. Also this section equates to my own experience of loss and bereavement, which is how I relate to what Thea is expressing here.

This note illustrates how my background, attitude and experiences shaped the research encounter that I had with Thea. Another researcher might not have asked this follow-up question, Thea might have recounted her story differently and my interpretation of her grief might have been ascribed to a different emotion. I asked myself to consider whether another couple, David and Victoria, who I had just interviewed had been somehow managing their emotions during the interview as they had been so articulate:

> I am mindful of only being able to ask people to express their emotions how they need to, or can. I am very conscious that my interviewing is flawed, however I am also pleased that, in this case at least, the couple have felt able to tell me quite a lot about their private thoughts. I think I have been very lucky to have had such a thoughtful couple to interview.

Another man, Andy, I had wrongly expected to be unable to express his feelings, and this assumption was based on my stereotyping as I was more comfortable at interviewing people more like me. The following observation is quite self-critical and painful to admit:

> Partly my prejudice was that Andy was not all that bright, a gym-fixated Neanderthal type man. Actually, I found myself realising that he's actually quite a thoughtful man and my assumptions about them as a couple (slightly bolshie, ignorant etc) were way off. They both surprised me and I feel quite ashamed of myself.

During the interview, I had with Cath and Andy (following their rearranged consultation) they provoke feelings of sadness in me and also I experience uncomfortable and conflicting emotions as I come to see the insider's perspective:

> As I am typing this I am struck again about how stream of consciousness this is. Both of them are wounded, they are really bewildered. I also continue to feel (myself) irritated by what they are saying, but also agreeing with it. I can't quite work out if I feel they don't deserve to be treated better because they don't pay lip service to the doctors or give them respect e.g. calling him 'that guy' or expecting a consultant to have phoned them up (As if! How Dickensian am I?!).

The tension I had here was to retain a researcher attitude rather than taking what the participants say as a personal attack on one of my other roles, as a clinic insider, in which I expected the doctor/patient roles as I knew them to be enacted. Of course, within the social setting of the clinic in the early twenty-first century these roles are not as defined as they once were and these participants' attitudes are completely normal. It was through reflecting on what these participants said that made me question my taken for granted assumptions about the setup and conduct of the medical encounters in the clinic. Andy had suggested that the consultant had been 'hard faced, angry and blunt' and that after:

> You know, the couple of years of trying, and all your friends getting pregnant and everybody asking you when are you going to have a baby and so there's a lot of emotion wrapped with it so you take all that emotion with you and you, you kind of want someone to be a little bit sympathetic.

A similar re-evaluation occurred during my interview with Katherine and William, a couple who had been due to start in vitro fertilisation (IVF) but had fallen pregnant naturally. They had chosen to use a private acupuncturist before starting the treatment, and attributed their pregnancy to this. My notes describe the confusion I felt during the interview, and I recognise this as stemming from again the tension between the insider-outsider perspectives, but also started my questioning of the biomedical model as the dominant authority of infertility. I reflected feeling:

> Strangely ambivalent about this interview. I am really happy for them but it seems amazingly lucky and I think part of me doesn't quite think they should be! But I am starting to doubt the medical aspect of this. I feel much as I did after seeing [X and Y] during Supervision. Perhaps there is something to this snake oil after all. My hackles rise at the presumption of the acupuncturist making clinical decisions, but there again why not? We are all shooting in the dark to some extent here.

At a later point in my research, during data analysis, these comments became very helpful in my findings around the role of the clinic and the patient in the pursuit of treatments for infertility.

Strategies for Reflexivity in the Field

Now that time has passed since the fieldwork stage of my thesis I have been able to reflect on what actually doing reflexivity entailed. I confess to not taking enough heed of this when I had read other researcher's accounts of their ethnographic and observational research. Descriptions of choosing notebooks, making snatched recordings in the sluice and wearing (or not) of uniforms seemed, before I entered the field myself, to be self-evident and the concerns with researcher attitude and emotions somewhat overstated. Now I consider the experiential learning of my observational fieldwork to have given me a revised perspective and with it strategies which I will utilise in my future research projects.

- Make a self-conscious decision to be a reflexive practitioner and to always use diaries and field notes in this pursuit at every research encounter. I found a recording device the most useful way of making short notes in this way.
- Acknowledge the complexities of being a professional who is also a researcher and the difficulties of managing dual identities.
- Don't underestimate the importance of supervision (or other review occasions) as an opportunity for support and debriefing, as well as appraisal.
- Finally, use emotional self-care strategies to provide some perspective when the 'swamp' threatens to overwhelm. These can be cognitive techniques such as meditation or distraction through physical exercise and focus on own time.

Conclusions

Research in 'human science', by its very nature, involves feelings and emotions, and the researcher cannot help but be caught up by this. Emotion work is closely linked to emotional intelligence and both demand qualities, such as self-awareness, empathy, warmth and sensitivity towards others, which enhance human relationships and therefore research encounters with people. Emotions are part of who we are, and help shape the social interactions through which understandings are formed and as qualitative research is largely about this knowledge, it cannot be separated from it. Indeed, being detached, and by implication, unemotional, are not attitudes that qualitative researchers should aspire to or cultivate. Without a doubt the emotion work in my study, and its impact on my understanding of my participants' experiences, was important and contributed significantly to the development of the findings in the thesis. Very few text books provide guidance on how to handle the emotions that are engendered when carrying out research or how to manage those emotions that arise when the private and professional selves clash (Cain, 2012).

Notes

1. Although in itself this argument presupposes that cultural groups are themselves open or closed and therefore to be understood differently by insiders and outsiders.
2. All participants have been given pseudonyms.
3. As it happens the following year Victoria, David and I met unexpectedly at a social event through a mutual friend. I think all of us enjoyed meeting up again in a different context, and but it did alter the dynamics of the event for me and I suspect that for them it must have been like being at a party with your accountant or priest. When we were chatting I was careful not to allude to the past (or indicate to anyone else our relationship) but Victoria did take five minutes ('as an aside') to tell me her latest news. They had found a suitable egg donor, which is a different outcome to their story than I had expected.

References

Allan, H. T. (1997). Reflexivity: A comment on feminist ethnography. *Journal of Research in Nursing, 2*(6), 455–467.

Allen, D. (2004). Ethnomethodological insights into insider-outsider relationships. *Nursing Inquiry, 11*(1), 14–24.

Arber, A. (2006). Reflexivity: A challenge for the researcher as practitioner? *Journal of Research in Nursing, 11*(2), 147–157.

Brewer, J. D. (2000). *Ethnography*. Buckingham: Open University Press.

Brocki, J., & Wearden, A. (2006). A critical evaluation of the use of interpretative phenomenological analysis (IPA) in health psychology. *Psychology and Health, 21*(1), 87–108.

Bryman, A. (1984). The debate about quantitative and qualitative research: A question of method or epistemology. *British Journal of Sociology, 35*(1), 75–92.

Cain, C. L. (2012). Emotions and the research interview: What hospice workers can teach us. *Health Sociology Review, 21*(4), 396–405.

Coffey, A. (1999). *The ethnographic self: Fieldwork and the representation of identity*. London; Thousand Oaks, CA: Sage.

Collington, V., & Hunt, S. C. (2006). Reflection in midwifery education and practice: An exploratory analysis. *Evidence Based Midwifery, 4*(3), 76–82.

Dickson-Swift, V., James, E. L., Kippen, S., & Liamputtong, P. (2008). Risk to researchers in qualitative research on sensitive topics: Issues and strategies. *Qualitative Health Research, 18*(1), 133–144. https://doi.org/10.1177/1049732307309007

Dickson-Swift, V., James, E. L., Kippen, S., & Liamputtong, P. (2009). Researching sensitive topics: Qualitative research as emotion work. *Qualitative Research, 9*, 61–79.

Duncombe, J., & Jessop, J. (2002). 'Doing rapport' and the ethics of 'faking friendship. In M. L. Mauthner, M. Birch, J. Jessop, & T. Miller (Eds.), *Ethics in qualitative research* (pp. 107–122). London: Sage.

Finaly, L. (1998). Reflexivity: An essential component for all research? *British Journal of Occupational Therapy, 61*, 453–456.

Finlay, L. (2002a). Negotiating the swamp: The opportunity and challenge of reflexivity in research practice. *Qualitative Research, 2*, 209–228.

Finlay, L. (2002b). "Outing" the researcher: The provenance, process, and practice of reflexivity. *Qualitative Health Research, 12*(4), 531–545.

Finlay, L. (2008). Reflecting on 'Reflective practice'. *PBPL paper 52* (p. 25). The Open University.

Fontana, A. (2004). Postmodern ethnography. In M. S. Lewis-Beck, A. Bryman, & T. F. Liao (Eds.), *The Sage encyclopedia of social science research methods*. Thousand Oaks, CA: Sage.

Froggatt, K. A. (1995). *Keeping the balance: Hospice work, death and emotions.* PhD doctoral, London South Bank University.

Greil, A. L., Slauson-Blevins, K., & McQuillan, J. (2010). The experience of infertility: A review of recent literature. *Sociology of Health & Illness, 32*(1), 140–162. https://doi.org/10.1111/j.1467-9566.2009.01213.x

Hammersley, M. (2013). *What's wrong with ethnography?* London: Routledge.
Hammersley, M., & Atkinson, P. (2007). *Ethnography: Principles in practice* (3rd ed.). London: Routledge.
Hedican, E. J. (2008). Empathy. In L. M. Given (Ed.), *The Sage encyclopedia of qualitative research methods* (p. 253). Los Angeles, CA; London: Sage.
Hochschild, A. R. (1983). *The managed heart: Commercialization of human feeling*. Berkeley; London: University of California Press.
Holloway, I., & Galvin, K. (2017). *Qualitative research in nursing and healthcare* (4th ed.). Chichester: Wiley & Sons.
Hunter, B. (2001). Emotion work in midwifery: A review of current knowledge. *Journal of Advanced Nursing, 34*(4), 436–444.
Hunter, B., & Deery, R. (2009). *Emotions in midwifery and reproduction.* Basingstoke: Palgrave Macmillan.
Jones, B., & Ficklin, L. (2012). To walk in their shoes: Recognising the expression of empathy as a research reality. *Emotion Space and Society, 5*(2), 103–112.
Koch, T. (1996). Implementation of a hermeneutic inquiry in nursing: Philosophy, rigour and representation. *Journal of Advanced Nursing, 24*(1), 174–184.
Lee-Treweek, G., & Linkogle, S. (2000). *Danger in the field: Risk and ethics in social research.* London; New York: Routledge.
Letherby, G. (2000). Dangerous liaisons: Auto/biography in research and research writing. In G. Lee-Treweek & S. Linkogle (Eds.), *Danger in the field: Risk and ethics in social research* (pp. 91–113). London; New York: Routledge.
Lipson, J. G. (1991). The use of self in ethnographic research. In J. M. Morse (Ed.), *Qualitative nursing research: A contemporary dialogue* (pp. 73–89). London: Sage.
Mackintosh, C. (2007). Protecting the self: A descriptive qualitative exploration of how registered nurses cope with working in surgical areas. *International Journal of Nursing Studies, 44*(6), 982–990. https://doi.org/10.1016/j.ijnurstu.2006.04.009
Maynard, M. (1994). Methods, practice and epistemology: The debate about feminism and research. In M. Maynard & J. Purvis (Eds.), *Researching women's lives from a feminist perspective* (pp. 10–27). London: Taylor & Francis.
McLeod, S. A. (2009). Emotion focused coping. Retrieved March 8, 2017, from http://www.simplypsychology.org/stress-management.html#em
Merleau-Ponty, M. (1962). *Phenomenology of perception* (C. Smith, Trans.). London: Routledge & Kegan Paul.
Pellatt, G. (2003). Ethnography and reflexivity: Emotions and feelings in fieldwork. *Nurse Researcher, 10*(3), 28–37. https://doi.org/10.7748/nr2003.04.10.3.28.c5894

Pelto, P. J. (2016). *Applied ethnography: Guidelines for field research*. London: Routledge.
Pillow, W. (2003). Confession, catharsis, or cure? Rethinking the uses of reflexivity as methodological power in qualitative research. *International Journal of Qualitative Studies in Education, 16*, 175–196.
Porter, S. (2000). Qualitative research. In D. Cormack (Ed.), *The research process in nursing* (4th ed., pp. 141–151). Oxford: Blackwell Science.
Rowling, L. (1999). Being in, being out, being with: Affect and the role of the qualitative researcher in loss and grief research. *Mortality, 4*(2), 167–181.
Schön, D. A. (1983). *The reflective practitioner: How professionals think in action*. New York: Basic Books.
Van Manen, M. (1990). *Researching lived experience: Human science for an action sensitive pedagogy*. London, ON: Althouse.
Watts, J. H. (2007). Emotion, empathy and exit: Reflections on doing ethnographic qualitative research on sensitive topics. *Medical Sociology Online, 3*(2), 3–14.
Williams, A. (1990). *Reflections on the making of an ethnographic text*. Studies in sexual politics, No. 29. Manchester: Manchester University Press.

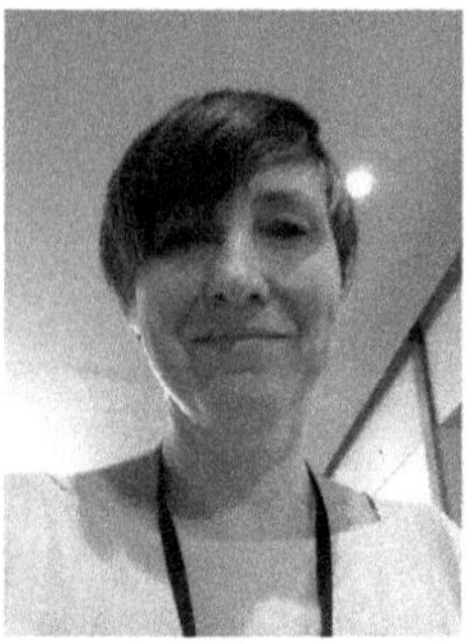

Ginny Mounce is a research midwife at Nuffield Department of Obstetrics and Gynaecology, University of Oxford, UK. She was awarded her Ph.D. in 2017 from the University of Surrey.

9

Pulling it All Together: Emotional Reflexivity in Health and Social Care Field Research

Helen T. Allan, Anne Arber, Nicola Ayers, Tam Chipawe Cane, Sarah Li, Ginny Mounce, and Kit Tapson

All the contributors to this book recommend taking a self-conscious decision to use emotional reflexivity as part of their research practice. Much thought has gone in to what it means to do reflexivity and what it means to be

H.T. Allan (✉)
Department of Adult, Child, Midwifery, Middlesex University, London, UK

A. Arber
University of Surrey, Guildford, UK

N. Ayers
Clinical Directorate, Federal Ministry of Health, Addis Ababa, Ethiopia

T.C. Cane
Department of Psychology, Social Work and Counselling, University of Greenwich, London, UK

S. Li
St George's, University of London, London, UK

G. Mounce
Nuffield Department of Obstetrics and Gynaecology, University of Oxford, Oxford, UK

K. Tapson
Centre for Arts as Wellbeing, University of Winchester, Winchester, UK

H.T. Allan, A. Arber (eds.), *Emotions and reflexivity in Health and Social Care Field Research*, https://doi.org/10.1007/978-3-319-65503-1_9

transparent about the goings-on in the field. This is important as roles such as researcher practitioner can impact on the research, especially where practice and research roles collide and influence the data collected. Having ways to step back and to reflect on subjectivities in practice and research enables an analytic eye on our own reactions as practitioners and researchers and these can be written in to methodologial accounts of the research.

Clearly at times, there were uncomfortable moments when questions were asked about who we were in relation to the research which led to discomfort and blurring of boundaries between research and practice. There were times when we identified with patients sharing the same condition as the people we were researching and mirroring their emotions in ourselves. Medical culture at times can appear over-harsh, especially when we straddle the professional, researcher and patient categories, and become a part of or witness to some distressing moments. Patients and clients can be categorised and judged as less worthy of access to services and empathy compared to others. Our feelings from witnessing these events then can cause difficulty when it comes to analysing and interpreting the data.

Research requires flexibility of thought and feeling as well as the emotion work to access the field, remain in the field and eventually leave the field in one way or another. This book identifies the lack of attention to support networks when out in the field for the researcher and also to the lack of awareness of supervisors of how field experiences impact on the research. This situation was not because academic and clinical supervisors were insensitive but researchers can be loath to report their field experiences or what they are dealing with in their research. This may be because many accounts of research are sanitised and tidy and written as non-problematic, lacking reflexive accounts of the research. Therefore, researchers can be out there in the field with precious little support to safely complete the research and leave the field unscathed. However, good practice regarding reflexivity and emotions are evident in our accounts, such as peer support, unburdening oneself in diary writing and journaling, and attentive supervisors and mentors.

In this book, the ups and downs of research, such as feeling high when things are going well and then alone and isolated from others when we run in to trouble, generate questions about how to manage and seek the right support at the right time. A thread running through the chapters is how the emotions in the field were at times overwhelming and the dilemmas around the research identity puzzling and complex. In many cases, emotions overwhelmed careful preparations and time out from the research was needed for balancing emotions and well-being. Using tools and strategies to do reflexivity and starting early on in the research process can help. Hearing people talk about their research experiences and contributing to such discussion in academic conferences can also help. Also taking time to read papers on reflexivity early on, perhaps at the same time as choosing a research design and thinking about methodology. Fabricius (1995) talks about adopting the 'third' position by which she means, reflecting-in-action (similar to Schon, 1983) through observing your feelings and reactions during the research. This could be practised in a safer situation than the field, perhaps with your supervisor or other research networks and moving forward from this being aware of how we position ourselves in the field and how we are positioned by others is an important aspect of reflexivity.

Several of the contributors have suggested that they would think about the supervisory relationship differently. Supervision contact may be a time (perhaps the only time) where the student feels their researcher role, issues in the field and experiences are understood. A few of us felt quite isolated during the research adopting, for example, a new role as a researcher within a workplace where one was known but also feeling confused and sometimes isolated about how to carry off the role (Chap. 8). One way that supervisors can be alert to how the fieldwork is progressing is through reading the research data which can highlight the identities adopted in the field and this can lead to further discussion about 'going native' as discussed in Chap. 7. We would recommend that close attention to transcripts of data, fieldnotes and research diaries can alert us to how the different identities manifest in the field, and this can lead to further discussion, analysis and support encouraging the turn to reflexivity. Facilitating emotional reflexivity through supervision opens up a lens through which new ideas and meaning making can emerge. Making a self-conscious decision to be a reflexive researcher and to use a research diary to record the researcher was helpful. Using an audio recorder on the way home from fieldwork was a good way to document and process field experiences. Coping with rejection during research was extremely difficult but offloading difficult emotional reactions in to the research diary allowed for catharsis (Chap. 2).

Emotional reflexivity allows the possibility to be creative and expressive to document the inevitable ups and downs, and this can be shared with others and written into methodological chapters. Perhaps unsurprisingly then, we recommend to keep a research journal/diary to facilitate emotional reflexivity. Such a diary or journal would document the researcher's thoughts, feelings and emotions, enable the researcher to remain cognisant of how the field and relationships in the field shape the researcher and the research. Keeping a journal also enables the researcher as an embodied presence to be present in the research, and this can add to credibility and transparency when writing up the research. We can also keep track of our methodological and theoretical assumptions and how these are both developed and experienced in the field.

Many of the chapters discuss researcher identity. Having dual, triple or multiple identities as a practitioner, researcher, counsellor, patient, can be not only advantageous but also problematic. Further blurring of boundaries can occur when research is carried out in one's workplace. Being a counsellor facilitated a safe space (Chap. 6) in which participants felt able to communicate their fragility, but research has time limitations and ethical boundaries. Synthesising our many identities is challenging, and keeping a marginal positioning can be difficult but of course using practices of reflection can alert us as to where we are at different moments and a record of such moments documented and made available for later interpretation (Chap. 4).

Another thread running through these chapters is the sensitive content of the field. Undertaking sensitive research with vulnerable participants, whether they're HIV positive, young people who bully, infertile couples or people who are dying, exposes the researcher to emotional risk. Finding ways to deal with this either through clinical supervision, academic supervision or counselling was essential. One of the contributors described how she used emotional self-care strategies to provide some perspective when the 'swamp' of the field threatened to overwhelm her. Examples of self-care strategies include cognitive techniques, such as meditation or distraction, physical exercise or just a focus on own time away from the field. Facilitating alternative support to address emotional disturbance and emotional burden or burnout may be necessary and clinical supervision should be considered alongside academic supervision. A secure virtual online supervisory space (discussion board perhaps) and SKYPE sessions especially when the researcher is abroad are required. Supervisors should also facilitate a safe space to 'empty out' anxieties or distress. Somewhere is needed for researchers to keep in touch with their supervisors during fieldwork to bridge the gap between a difficult interview or observation and the next scheduled supervision session. Researchers should also feel able to approach their supervisors about their emotional well-being and anxieties without worrying about placing a potential burden on supervisors.

It is important to know your research community and how to manage research located in a 'small world'. Indeed, 'culturally' appropriate communication should not be limited to language but include preparing oneself to communicate sensitively and appropriately with participants from many communities. Working with vulnerable participants requires additional thought and emotional management skills: to be aware of using evaluating words, for example, or over-identifying with participants as caring or non-caring. Being a researcher amongst vulnerable participants may include feelings of discomfort. It helpful to be reflexively aware of this discomfort and embrace the situation and learn through it. This then allowed the 'shared emotional space' to develop from which flowed good data. Recording in the journal or diary pre-existing judgements and misconceptions to reduce the impact they could have on the research is helpful. It is important that researchers clarify their own a priori conceptions to facilitate the reflexive process. Clearly identifying unique experiences and mapping out similarities and differences in experiences between participants and the researcher would enable openness and transparency to written accounts of fieldwork.

Emotions in the field arise from both the researcher themselves, the topic of the research and the field relationships and interactions, and these should encourage and motivate us towards a reflexivity which includes emotions.

As a result of writing this book and bringing the different chapters together, we suggest:

- Record thoughts and feelings about field experiences in the diary or journal include the uncomfortable feelings and discuss them in supervision
- Be intuitive—respond to bodily feelings and note them in your research journal or diary
- Build a good research network with academic peers and use this network to talk about the ups and downs of research and to receive peer support
- Supervisors—allow some space, mental and emotional, for de-briefing maintain a listening space for researchers to talk about their emotions and field experiences
- Supervisors should encourage the reflexive researcher to write themselves in and this adds to the credibility of the research account

We argue that emotional reflexivity should not be temporary or inconsistent but an on-going process at all stages of the research from planning to publication and thoughts and feelings to actions. We have suggested that there is a broader need within Academia to consider emotional reflexivity in field research as an important aspect at all stages of the research journey and an important part of the natural history of field research.

References

Fabricius, J. (1995). Psychoanalytic understanding and nursing: A supervisory workshop with nurse tutors. *Psychoanalytic Psychotherapy, 9*, 17–29.

Schon, D. (1983). *The reflective practitioner: How professionals think in action.* London: Temple Smith.

Helen T. Allan is Professor in Nursing at the Centre for Critical Research in Nursing & Midwifery, Middlesex University, London, UK. Helen was awarded her Ph.D. in 2000 from the Royal College of Nursing Institute/University of Manchester. Helen has supervised Ph.D. and clinical doctorates since 2002.

Anne Arber is Senior Lecturer in Cancer and Palliative Care, School of Health Sciences, University of Surrey, Guildford, Surrey, UK. Anne was awarded her Ph.D. in 2004 from Goldsmiths, University of London, UK. Anne conducts research in cancer and palliative care. She has supervised Ph.D. and clinical doctorate students since 2004.

Nicola Ayers is Palliative Care Advisor in the Clinical Directorate, Federal Ministry of Health, Ethiopia. She was awarded her Ph.D. from the University of Surrey in 2015.

Tam Chipawe Cane is Senior Lecturer, Programme Leader for Social Work Programmes at the University of Greenwich, UK. She was awarded her clinical doctorate from the University of Surrey in 2015.

Sarah Li is an honorary research fellow at Kingston University and St George's, University of London, Faculty of Health, Social Care & Wellbeing, UK. Sarah has conducted research in palliative care, mental health and care of older people. She was awarded her Ph.D. in 2002 from Goldsmiths, University of London.

Ginny Mounce is a research midwife at Nuffield Department of Obstetrics and Gynaecology, University of Oxford, UK. She was awarded her Ph.D. in 2017 from the University of Surrey.

Kit Tapson is a research fellow at the Centre for Arts and Wellbeing, University of Winchester, UK. She was awarded her clinical doctorate from the University of Surrey in 2015.

Index

H.T. Allan, A. Arber (eds.), *Emotions and reflexivity in Health and Social Care Field Research*, https://doi.org/10.1007/978-3-319-65503-1

CPI Antony Rowe
Chippenham, UK
2019-09-13 13:14